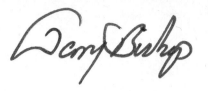

Clinical neurology

F   Ess. 2001
NO REFUND IF LABEL IS REMOVED
N. Y. U. BOOK CENTER
DO $11.45⁑

Clinical neurology

FRANCIS M. FORSTER, B.S., M.D.

Professor and Chairman, Department of Neurology,
University of Wisconsin School of Medicine,
Madison, Wisconsin

FOURTH EDITION

The C. V. Mosby Company

Saint Louis   1978

FOURTH EDITION

Copyright © 1978 by The C. V. Mosby Company

All rights reserved. No part of this book may be reproduced
in any manner without written permission of the publisher.

Previous editions copyrighted 1962, 1966, 1973

Printed in the United States of America

The C. V. Mosby Company
11830 Westline Industrial Drive, St. Louis, Missouri 63141

Library of Congress Cataloging in Publication Data

Forster, Francis M
  Clinical neurology.

  Bibliography: p.
  Includes index.
  1. Nervous system—Diseases. 2. Neurology.
I. Title. [DNLM: 1. Nervous system diseases.
WL100 F733s]
RC356.F6 1978   616.8   78-7343
ISBN 0-8016-1637-9

C/CB/CB 9 8 7 6 5 4 3 2 1

TO
B.V.M.H.

PREFACE

This book was first published in 1962. The purpose of the volume through these years has been to present the methodologies used in making an evaluation of the neurologic patient and the most significant features of the diseases in the field of clinical neurology. The presentation has been based on clarity and brevity, with emphasis on categories relative to their importance. Therefore the clinical entities occurring relatively infrequently have been set in reduced type.

Neurology can be a confusing field with a cluttering of eponyms. These eponyms have therefore been reduced to a minimum, and when these terms have been used, they usually have been included as parenthetical names.

This book was designed primarily for medical students as a primer when they begin their clinical work. It has also been found to be of extensive use in the paramedical field for nurses, occupational therapists, physical therapists, pharmacy students, social workers, rehabilitation counselors, various laboratory personnel, including EEG technicians, and various psychology students and technicians.

Since the book is not meant to be encyclopedic by any manner or means, adequate pertinent references are appended to each chapter.

Francis M. Forster

CONTENTS

PART ONE **EVALUATION OF THE NEUROLOGIC PATIENT**

1 The neurologic history

In taking a neurologic history physicians search diligently into the where, why, how, and when features of a patient's complaints. Obviously questions are guided by their knowledge of the type of disease suspected. This section serves to establish some guidelines in questioning techniques. The questions asked depend largely on familiarity with the syndromes and diseases described in later sections of the book.

FAMILY HISTORY

The physician is interested in documenting the presence of neurologic disorders in the forebears, collaterals, and siblings of the patient. The exact questioning frequently depends on the presenting complaint of the individual patient. For example, if the patient has seizures, one is interested in whether there were convulsions, spasms, or seizures in the parents, grandparents, great-grandparents, cousins, aunts, uncles, or other relations. One also needs to inquire regarding spasms occurring in childhood or in association with fever. If the disorder involves the cerebellum or basal ganglia and is suspected to be familial, again one must inquire specifically about relatives such as parents, grandparents, aunts, uncles, and cousins. Details of the family illnesses are necessary. In migraine, for example, one needs to know the type of headache present in the family—not merely that headaches occurred.

PAST HISTORY

In inquiring into the past history of neurologic patients, it is important to have in most instances a clear record of the **an-**

tenatal and **perinatal circumstances.** The exact place in birth order is important (and it is important also to include miscarriages and abortions, in their proper order). Among other factors are questions such as whether the mother was exposed to any infections or trauma during her pregnancy, whether the delivery was normal, whether forceps were used, whether the infant was able to leave the hospital at the same time as the mother, whether there was any concern regarding the baby's health after birth, and whether oxygen had to be used.

The **developmental history** must be carefully determined. At what ages did the child begin to walk and to talk? How did he compare with his siblings? How did he progress in nursery school, kindergarten, and later educational situations? What were his relationships with other children?

The **occurrence of previous illnesses** must be documented, including the usual childhood diseases. Complications of childhood diseases are significant, especially with the exanthems and with inoculations. Inquiries are made as to the severity of any illness such as pneumonia. The degree of hypoxia and the duration of high temperature assume neurologic significance.

The role of head injury is sometimes difficult to evaluate. Most children have experienced some minor head injuries. Severity of a head injury is indicated by resultant loss of consciousness, the presence or absence of posttraumatic symptoms, whether the severity led to consulting the family physician, and whether the patient required roentgenologic examination.

PRESENT ILLNESS

The **onset of the present illness** usually can be fixed with fair accuracy. In the neurologic analysis one generally can identify the time of onset. In weakness of one side of the body, for example, it may be the time at which the patient had to change his job habits or when he found it necessary to rest after walking a particular distance. In the case of posterior column disease, history can fix the time at which it became necessary to touch the washstand while washing the face with eyes closed.

The **chief complaint** must be exactly characterized. For example, in examining a patient with headache, the physician gives him a long list of characteristic descriptive terms (e.g., dull, throbbing, burning, pressing, stabbing, bandlike) and asks him to choose the appropriate term or terms. In episodic disturbances of the nervous system, the duration of individual episodes should be carefully documented, the longest, shortest, and average durations being specified. Associated symptoms are of great importance when disorders are episodic. The first interview is the ideal time to determine the usual frequency, as well as the shortest and longest time intervals between episodes. To document this accurately, the physician should record the times of the most recent episodes.

When a symptom is steadily progressive, it is often possible to obtain definitive **evidence of the progression.** For example, in weakness of one side of the body, some point can be established, such as the time when the patient could no longer walk a particular distance—like four blocks—or climb stairs or when the upper extremities could last be used in activities such as typing, playing the piano, or lighting a cigarette. Thus indications of progression or improvement are derived.

In all complaints the presence or absence of **precipitating factors** is ascertained. Precipitating factors play an important role, for example, in the rupture of cerebral aneurysms. Engaging in coitus or straining at stool often precipitates the symptoms of an existing aneurysm. When a patient with a brain tumor suffers sudden loss of consciousness after expelling an enema, the circumstance is highly suggestive of brain herniation at the foramen magnum and at the tentorium. In some cases of epilepsy, the quest for precipitating factors elicits those rare and unusual musicogenic epilepsies or startle epilepsies. In certain facial pain syndromes the precipitation by chewing or swallowing suggests immediately a glossopharyngeal neuralgia.

The **condition of the patient at the onset of the neurologic dis-**

order becomes of great importance, particularly when an episode has a relatively acute period of onset. An abrupt onset is characteristic of vascular disease. When this occurs during a period of decreased activity such as sleeping, it is more likely to be due to an encephalomalacia, whereas occurrence during a period of increased activity is more often found to be of hemorrhagic nature. In some of the rare central nervous system manifestations, posture also becomes important; for example, in carotid sinus syncope the attacks occur only when the individual is in a sitting or a standing position. In hypoglycemic attacks the importance of time relationship to food intake is obvious.

REVIEW OF SYSTEMS

A careful review of systems may give clues not only to the primary disease of the nervous system but also to general systemic diseases that may be causing the neurologic manifestations. With the neurologic patient therefore the physician is particularly careful to query the review of systems in regard to vision for such indications as the presence of blurring of vision, diplopia, or oscillopsia (visual awareness of nystagmus by the patient). These may be suggestive of multiple sclerosis. Hemianopsia occurs in the vascular types of headache. Evaluation of the eighth cranial nerve shows that tinnitus, progressive loss of hearing, and vertigo occur with lesions of this nerve—either neoplastic in nature or due to Meniere's disease.

A history of chronic severe upper respiratory infections such as mastoiditis or sinusitis may indicate the possible existence of brain abscess or meningitis. The presence of cough, wasting, weight loss, and night sweats raises the possibility of tuberculosis or carcinoma of the lung.

Dyspnea, tachycardia, and ankle edema, of course, point to cardiovascular disease and it concomitant effect on the cerebral circulation.

The presence of gastroenteric symptoms may suggest the

influence of a cerebral lesion on that system or, more commonly, the metastasis of a neoplasm of the gastroenteric tract to the central nervous system.

Review of the genitourinary tract symptoms may indicate a lesion that perhaps has spread to the nervous system, or it may give evidence of primary central nervous system involvement. Carcinomas, especially of the prostate, metastasize to the vertebral bodies. Tumors of the adrenal glands and kidneys, particularly hypernephromas, may metastasize widely to the central nervous system. Lesions of the central nervous system may produce retention of urine or urinary incontinence and, particularly in men, impairment of libido and potency.

In the **general review,** it is important to determine (1) if the patient has been exposed to toxic agents such as alcohol, heavy metals, or carbon monoxide; (2) whether his nutrition, including vitamin intake, has been adequate; (3) what preceding infections the patient has had and the therapy used therefore; and (4) what traumatic episode the patient has experienced, particularly in relationship to the disease entity, for example, head injuries in epileptics or back injuries in patients with lumbar disk syndromes.

It is not possible to formulate the detailed and precise manner of taking a history, since this varies with each individual patient. It depends on the nature of the illness that has brought the patient to the physician, on the patient's accuracy as a witness and his ability to communicate, and most important of all, on the physician's willingness to spend the time to search diligently and carefully and in a nonsuggestive way. It is always important to present the patient with multiple choices or descriptions so as to avoid putting words into his mouth. In history taking, the need for other witnesses, such as relatives and co-workers, is obvious.

Considerable skill must be developed in obtaining a patient's history. The mere putting down on paper of the recollections of the patient is not appropriate. The facts not only must be assembled but they also must be organized. In the acquisition of facts, skill is necessary to direct the patient away from irrelevant musings but still pay attention to trivia. One of the physician's most important decisions concerns what is present illness and what is past history. The determination as to whether the chief complaint is part of a continuing illness or is a separate entity is an indication of the diagnostic process. Too often significant facts gathered by medical students and house staff are overlooked because in the organization of the material not enough emphasis was placed on what appeared to be an obscure fact.

Competent neurologists expect by way of the history to arrive at a reasonable differential diagnosis. The physical and neurologic examinations usually succeed in decreasing the choices in the differential diagnosis, and the laboratory is used to make the final discrimination between the two or three most likely alternatives. This is the most logical way to arrive at neurologic diagnoses. Most neurologists, when the history leaves them at sea, are extremely uncomfortable about the possibility of being unable to arrive at an adequate and competent diagnosis even after the detailed examination.

2 The neurologic examination

The neurologic examination of the conscious patient requires more patient participation than that required in other types of medical examinations. Therefore this puts a premium on the communication between physician and patient. The demonstration by the physician of what is wanted should accompany the command. For example, the examiner extends his own arms and abducts his fingers when he says, "Hold out your arms and spread your fingers." Sometimes other modalities of learning are also used. The command, given only, "Put your heel on your knee" is perplexing. The command should be accompanied by a light touch to one heel at the word "heel" and to the opposite knee at the word "knee." These simple techniques not only obtain improved patient participation and a smoothness of the examination but also heighten the patient's confidence in the examiner.

EXAMINATION OF STATION AND GAIT

If the patient is ambulatory, examination of the station and gait is usually performed at the beginning of the neurologic examination.

Station is tested by having the patient stand with feet closely apposed to each other, both heel and toe, first with the eyes open and then with them closed. A positive Romberg sign consists of marked swaying and falling when the eyes are closed. The patient is then instructed to open his eyes and to stand on one foot alone and then on the other so that the station is tested for each foot individually.

Gait is observed in the patient's usual walking pattern. The patient is next asked to walk on his heels, then to walk on his toes, and finally to walk tandem, that is, apposing the heel on one foot to the toe of the other and continuing in this fashion—walking the "straight and narrow." These tests not only bring out **equilibration** but also are indications of **motor power** in the lower extremities. This can be tested further by having the patient squat and rise and then squat and duck walk.

EXAMINATION OF THE CRANIUM

The scalp is inspected for evidences of **injury,** both recent (such as hematomas) and remote (such as scars), for **congenital lesions,** particularly the hemangiomas, and for the presence of moles.

The cranium is inspected for **dyssymmetry** and is palpated to determine whether there are any **exostoses,** areas of tenderness, or depression of the skull. The cranium is auscerted for **bruits,** the most common places being over the temporal and frontal areas and over the orbit; also included is any likely spot indicated by history or other findings as the possible site of neoplasm or vascular malformation. At this point it is customary, in addition, to auscult the **carotid arteries** for bruits not transmitted from the heart and to palpate for the pulsations of the carotid arteries.

EXAMINATION OF THE CRANIAL NERVES

The **first cranial nerve** can be simply tested by using a piece of perfumed soap. The identification of perfume indicates that there is no anosmia.

The **second cranial nerve** is examined by direct funduscopy with observation for the clarity of the disk edges, presence of the cup, caliber of the veins, and evidence of exudate or hemorrhages. Alterations of these indicate papilledema or optic neuritis. Pallor of the disk indicates optic atrophy. The physician must be careful not to be misled by a normal difference between the nasal and temporal edges of the disk, the temporal normally being more sharply defined than the nasal edge. The maculas are inspected. Particularly in children who may have degenerative diseases, it is important to determine that there is no pigmentary degeneration of the maculas. It is also necessary to scan the peripheral areas of the retinas for lesions such as retinitis pigmentosa, chorioretinitis of toxoplasma, tuberculomas, or small petechial hemorrhages.

In older patients the condition of the retinal vessels may be a clue to the vascular status. Also in patients suspected of cerebrovascular disease, a careful search after pupillary dilatation may reveal emboli that are either thrombin or cholesterol in content.

The optic nerve is also examined by the determination of peripheral visual fields. This can be done by having the patient close one eye while the examiner closes his own opposite eye and then brings in his fingers from the side, holding his hands equidistant between the patient and himself. In this way he compares his own visual field with those of the patient. With a little experience it is possible for the examiner to determine macular fields also by becoming aware of the point at which his own finger is not perceived merely as blurred movement but is readily apparent as a finger. This marks his own macular field.

With children and patients who cannot cooperate well, the physician will forego these computations. Examination of the visual fields can then be accomplished by asking the patient to identify the number or location of rapidly flicking fingers in the peripheral fields or noting when attention is attracted by shiny objects introduced laterally in the field. It is possible to determine scotomas by using a dark-headed corsage pin against a white examining coat, having the patient look at a button of the coat and tell when the corsage pin disappears. Visual acuity can be crudely tested by using the various headlines of a newspaper and again comparing the examiner's acuity (of which he is usually well aware) with that of the patient.

More detailed examinations of visual fields, of course, are necessary for careful patient records, and these can be done on the perimeter, tangent screen, or stereocampimeter (Chapter

3). In general, neurologists prefer the tangent screen to all other devices. It provides not only a good outline of the peripheral field but also an excellent opportunity for mapping scotomas and for repeated studies of a scotoma of any size.

Examination of the **third, fourth,** and **sixth cranial nerves** includes noting the pupillary size, regularity, reaction to light, and accommodation. It is important not to hold the flashlight so that it shines directly into the eyes when studying the light reflex, since the patient may then accommodate to the light, and the examiner in that case would be testing both reaction to light and accommodation. External ocular movements are tested by having the patient look at a small object, the head of a corsage pin again being ideal. One must be certain that this is in contrast with the background, such as a light pin against a dark background or a dark pin against a light background. A small object is necessary to bring out nystagmus of slight degree. The test object is carried to one side and then to the other, next is moved up and down, and then is brought in for convergence.

If there is some question of impaired convergence, it is best to have the patient look out the window at an object across the street and then at the test object held a few inches from his nose. The extent of extraocular movement in all phases is carefully noted for impairment; the patient is often the best witness of this by his indicating the appearance of diplopia.

Determination of the involvement causing the diplopia can be made by placing a red lens in front of one eye and finding out which image is red and which is not red, thus mapping or distinguishing the false image from the true. Another simple way is to use a reflex hammer as the test object and to give the patient another reflex hammer to place over the false image. This will also give the direction of the diplopia—whether it is parallel or oblique. Horizontal parallel diplopia occurs with lesions of either the internal or external rectus muscle. Since the external rectus has a single nerve supply, this is the one most commonly involved. All other muscle impairments give an oblique type of diplopia.

At this point nystagmus also is carefully observed. This may be horizontal, vertical, or rotary. As noted previously, it is important to use a small test object to detect nystagmus, particularly when it is of slight degree. Therefore use of the corsage pin is recommended. In determining the type of nystagmus, it is much simpler to look at a dichotomy of a small blood vessel in the sclera and to follow this for direction rather than to attempt to look at the entire cornea. When nystagmus is questionable, as to either presence or range, the physician may have the patient fix his eyes on a small object in the direction in which the questionable nystagmus was elicited and may then observe the fundus. The magnification of the ophthalmoscope, of course, enlarges the range of the nystagmus and makes it simpler to determine whether there is a rotary or a vertical component.

The sensory examination of the **fifth cranial nerve** is usually omitted at this point and postponed until the total sensory examination is carried out later, but at the time of testing eye movements the corneal reflexes are tested. Again the test object is carried to the side, usually somewhat upward so that the eyes are in a lateral and upward gaze, and a wisp of cotton or a horsehair is touched briskly to the cornea at the limbus. It is important not to have the wisp of cotton or hair touch enough of the cornea so that it crosses the pupil, since then a visual defensive action is obtained rather than a sensory response from the cornea. The motor portion of the fifth cranial nerve is tested by having the patient chew while the examiner's fingers are placed on the masseters and the temporal muscles. Thus the quality of their functions is observed. The pterygoid muscles are tested by having the patient open his mouth widely. It is best to use the handle of a reflex hammer, sight from the bridge of the nose to the supraclavicular notch for fixed points, and measure any deviation from the plumb line of the reflex hammer, using the notch between the central incisors or the cleft of the lower jaw as the moving point to be sighted. The pterygoid muscles are further tested by having the patient forcibly move the jaw against the examiner's thumb, first to one side and then to the other.

In examining the **seventh cranial,** or **facial, nerve,** motor power of the upper part of the face is noted by comparing the two sides while having the patient first frown and then look surprised. The eyes are forcibly closed against resistance, and in this way the orbicularis oculi muscles are tested. Showing the teeth, smiling, and puckering the lips to whistle bring out weakness of the lower face.

The differentiation of peripheral (due to involvement of the seventh cranial nerve or its nucleus) from central (due to a lesion of the face area of the motor cortex or the corticobulbar tract) facial palsy is determined by the presence or absence of involvement of the upper portion of the face. If the lesion is peripheral, the entire motor distribution is involved. If a peripheral facial palsy is old, evidence of crossed regeneration can often be demonstrated. Rapid blinking of the eyes will, on the affected side, cause simultaneous small contractions of the orbicularis oris, and conversely, movements of the orbicularis oris will be accompanied by contractions of the orbicularis oculi.

When the need is indicated, taste can be tested in the following way: Put a few grains of salt on a tongue depressor, have the patient protrude the tongue, gently massage these grains into one side of the tongue (not allowing the patient to withdraw the tongue but telling him to indicate by holding up a finger when he has tasted something), and then have him identify the taste by nodding his head "yes" or "no" to each of the different types of taste mentioned.

In routine neurologic practice the **eighth cranial nerve** can be tested by using a tuning fork. This should be a 256-cycle fork, since a 128-cycle fork adds vibratory sensations that confuse the results of the test. For testing air conduction, the tuning fork is held near the pinna on one side, and the patient is asked to tell when the sound disappears as the tuning fork is carried laterally. At the point at which it disappears, the examiner's finger can be placed on the shoulder. Then the same test is done on the other side. Thus air conduction on the two sides can be rapidly compared. The relationship of air conduction to bone conduction is next tested by placing the tuning fork again in front of the ear and then over the mastoid process. The patient is asked to indicate which sound is louder. The tuning fork is then placed over the forehead in the midline, and the patient is asked if he hears it and, if so, where. The normal response is midline. Lateralization to either ear may be indicated by the patient.

Functions of the **ninth, tenth,** and **twelfth cranial nerves** are usually tested together. The patient is asked to protrude his tongue. Again deviation of the tongue can be measured with the handle of the reflex hammer, this time using the bridge of the nose and the cleft of the jaw as the sighting points and noting any deviation of the furrow of the tongue to one side or the other. The gag reflex is tested by touching the pharynx with a tongue blade and observing the quality of the reflex on the two sides. Phonation produces movement of the palate, and thus deviation of the palate can be determined. At this time voice is tested by asking the patient to count from one to ten, and speech is tested for slurring by having the patient repeat test phrases such as "Commonwealth of Pennsylvania," "Methodist Episcopal," and "around the rugged rock the ragged rascal ran." Scanning is best elicited by using either blank verse or a similar prose statement, such as "Fourscore and seven years ago our fathers," etc. The patient is asked to cough, and the presence or absence of a staccato type of cough is noted. Swallowing is observed at this time.

Functions of the **eleventh cranial nerve** are tested by asking the patient to rotate the head forcibly, first to one side and then to the other. In both instances the examiner resists the movement by placing one hand on the jaw, and with the other he palpates the sternomastoid muscle being tested. After this the examiner places his hands on the shoulders and requests the patient to shrug his shoulders against resistance.

EXAMINATION OF THE SPINE

The condition of the **cervical spine** is determined by flexing the neck, with fingers placed over the cervical spine, and noting the degree of mobility of the spine, the presence or absence of nuchal rigidity, a limitation of motion in any direction, and any crepitus due to arthritic change. Flexing the head may also bring out an unusual sign (Lhermitte's), in which the patient subjectively complains of a tingling, vibratory, or electric sensation down the spine or down the lower or upper extremities at the time of flexion of the head. When nuchal rigidity is present, the physician usually deviates at this time to test for Kernig's sign, obtained by flexing the thigh to 90 degrees and then extending the leg at the knee. A positive sign consists of limitation of extension at the knee. This sign, combined with nuchal rigidity, indicates meningeal irritation.

The mobility of the **lumbar spine** is noted in much the same way as that of the cervical spine, that is, by placing the fingers over the spinous processes during posterior, anterior, and lateral flexions of the spine.

Observation is used to determine whether there is any scoliosis or other abnormality of the spine. Tufting of the hair over the lumbosacral region indicates a possible anomaly (spina bifida occulta). The spinous processes are percussed with a reflex hammer to elicit local tenderness. In addition, forcible pressure may be exerted on the cranium to elicit local tenderness of the spine.

EXAMINATION OF THE UPPER EXTREMITIES

For examination of the upper extremities, the patient is instructed to extend his arms in space directly in front of him, spread his fingers widely, and close his eyes. Inspection at this time is for the purpose of determining **involuntary movements** or **abnormal postures** of the hands. Drifting of the upper extremities downward indicates weakness, whereas drifting to the side or upward indicates proprioceptive or cerebellar disturbance. Observation here is also concerned with evidence of **dyssymmetry of body parts.** Smallness of an extremity or a decrease in nipple to midsternal distance suggests a lesion of the opposite postcentral gyrus.

Inspection at this point is employed also to observe the **mus-**

cle status of the upper extremities for the existence of any focal atrophy or the presence of fasciculations. When fasciculations are particularly expected, the arms are again placed at rest after this slight exertion. The muscles of the shoulder girdle are then percussed briskly and observed for increased myotatic irritability. If relaxation after activity, plus the percussion, does not bring out fasciculations, gentle cool breathing on the part may elicit them.

With arms maintained in space and eyes closed, the patient is instructed to touch the tip of his nose with his finger, with each hand separately. After this, eyes are opened and the patient is instructed to touch the examiner's finger and then his own nose and to do this repeatedly and rapidly. The **cerebellar signs** of dyssynergia, dysmetria, and intention tremor can be observed at this point. Dyssynergia means improper working together of muscles so that a motor act which is made up of complex movements (such as touching finger to nose) is broken down into its parts. Dysmetria means a disturbance of measuring so that the patient does not properly measure the distances between his nose and the examiner's fingertip and will thus miss the tip, deviating to the right or the left or stopping short, or he will hit the fingertip too forcibly. Intention tremor is usually most obvious near the end of the act.

Dysrhythmia is tested by having the patient rapidly tap the hand of the examiner with his hand, palm to palm, or tap the floor with his foot. Any disturbance in the rhythm of the action is noted. Rebound phenomenon occurs when the patient forcibly flexes his arm at the elbow and the examiner suddenly releases the patient's arm. Muscle tone is evaluated by rapidly moving the extremity with the patient relaxed. Spasticity is evidenced by increased tone similar to that of the spring of a clasp knife. This is evident on passive extension of fingers, wrist, and elbow. After this, digital movements are tested by having the patient rapidly touch his thumb to the tip of each finger. Dexterity between the two sides is compared, not only for motor power but also for normal cerebellar function.

A detailed survey of **motor function** of the upper extremities includes handgrips compared bilaterally, usually tested objectively by having the patient squeeze the examiner's fingers. If an actual measurement is necessary, the dynamometer can be employed. The abduction and adduction of fingers, as well as their flexion and extension, apposition of the thumb to the little finger, flexion and extension at the wrist and elbow, elevation and depression of the humerus, abduction and adduction of the humerus to the chest, and forcible adduction of the extended arms—all give a brief survey of the appendicular and axial muscles of the upper extremities.

The most important deep tendon **reflexes** of the upper extremities are the biceps, the triceps, and the radial. The biceps reflex is elicited by placing the examiner's thumb over the biceps tendon with the arm in flexion and relaxation, the wrist being supported. The examiner's thumb is percussed with the reflex hammer. The triceps reflex is most critically obtained by having the arm abducted at the shoulder and hanging in flexion at the elbow. The degree of excursion of the arm on direct percussion of the triceps tendon can be observed. The radial reflex is obtained with the arms flexed and supported in the lap of the patient. The distal end of the radius is briskly percussed directly with the reflex hammer and the slight contraction of the brachioradialis noted. If any of these responses are hyperactive, there may even be repetitive responses or clonus.

The finger jerk is a useful reflex for determining differences between the tendon reflexes in the two upper extremities. To obtain this the examiner places his hand in pronation with his fingers flexed; then, with the patient's fingers flexed also and his hands supine, the examiner's fingers are placed in the palm of the patient's hand and gently tug against the patient's flexed fingers. The examiner then percusses his own fingers briskly with a reflex hammer. The test therefore makes possible not only the visual evaluation but also the examiner's own proprioceptive evaluation of the patient's reflex finger flexion.

Of the finger signs, the most important is the Hoffmann sign, which is obtained by flicking the nail of the third finger and watching for flexion and apposition of thumb and index finger. For best results the examiner clutches the patient's third finger between his own index and middle fingers with his thumb over the nail, gently shakes the patient's hand several times to obtain relaxation, and then quickly flicks the nail of the third finger.

In all reflex testing it should be emphasized that asymmetry of response is the most important observation.

EXAMINATION OF THE ABDOMEN

The state of the bladder is evaluated by palpating and percussing the bladder level. Abdominal reflexes are obtained by briskly stroking the abdomen with an object sharp enough to give noxious stimulation but not enough to break the surface of the skin. Each quadrant of the abdomen is stroked separately so that a diamond figure is drawn several inches away from the umbilicus. At each stroke the presence or absence of movement of the umbilicus toward the stimulated area is noted.

EXAMINATION OF THE LOWER EXTREMITIES

The **posture** of the lower extremities is examined by having the patient maintain his legs in space, with the eyes again closed and the two legs separated slightly so that neither one can support or guide the other. In this test also any drifting of the affected part is noted. Whenever a drift from slight weakness of one side is suspected, it can best be brought out by having the patient lie prone, with the knees flexed so that the legs are maintained in space again separately but just short of 90 degrees from the examining table. The hamstring tendons are gently percussed equally and bilaterally to obtain some relaxation, and then the posture of the leg is noted for a gradual drooping on the afflicted side.

After the evaluation of posture, **coordination** is tested by the heel-to-knee-to-shin test and the toe-to-object test. Since the heel-to-knee-to-shin test may show a pseudoataxia because of too firm a pressure of the heel on the shin, patients are instructed that this is to be done gently, smoothly, and expeditiously. Also proper draping of the patient is necessary to obtain a facile performance. The toe-to-object test is obtained by holding a finger or an object such as the reflex hammer in space at a point reasonable for the patient and instructing him to touch this object with his great toe, with his eyes open.

Motor power is tested by having the patient wiggle his toes, first on one side and then on the other, and comparing function on the two sides. Plantar and dorsal flexion of the ankle, flexion and extension at knee and hip, adduction and abduction of the hip, and internal and external rotation are tested, in that order.

The **muscle status** is observed for evidence of atrophy and for fasciculations.

The important tendon **reflexes** in the lower extremities are the patellar and the Achilles tendon reflexes. The former is obtained by direct percussion of the patellar tendon, infrapatellarly. A suprapatellar reflex is indicative of hyperactivity. The suprapatellar reflex is elicited by cupping the examiner's index finger over the patient's patella, gently tugging the patella downward, and then briskly percussing the examiner's finger. The Achilles reflex may be demonstrated when the legs are placed in a frog position (abduction and flexion of the hip and flexion at the knee), with the ankle dorsiflexed, and the Achilles tendon is briskly percussed. This reflex may also be obtained when the legs are extended and, with the examiner's hand placed over the volar surface of the foot, the hand of the examiner is percussed. In any of these maneuvers, for either the Achilles or the patellar reflex, clonus can be elicited and, of course, indicates hyperactive deep tendon reflexes. It is noteworthy, however, that in periods of extreme tension normal individuals may have ankle clonus.

The **plantar signs** are numerous, indeed myriad. The most important of these is the sign of Babinski. This sign is elicited by applying a noxious stimulus to the lateral plantar surface of the foot. The noxious stimulus should not be one that breaks the surface of the skin, but the practice of using some innocuous object, such as the end of a reflex hammer, is to be decried. Readily available instruments include an orange stick and the end of an open paper clip (it is important to be certain, however, that there is no burr at the end of the clip). Before the stimulus is applied, the patient should be relaxed and forewarned that his foot is to be scratched. The hip, knee, and ankle are gently flexed and the toes are gently massaged back and forth a few times until maximal relaxation is obtained. Then the noxious stimulus is applied far laterally on the sole of the foot over the heel and brought slowly upward toward the base of the little toe and then across to the base of the great toe. Normally all the toes curl in plantar flexion. The positive sign is the tonic, gradual, almost majestic dorsiflexion of the great toe, usually accompanied by flaring of the lesser digits. There are certain other minor components of the reflex, such as contraction of the tensor fascia lata, but by and large it is the movement of the great toe that is the hallmark of this sign.

Chaddock's sign is evidenced by dorsiflexion of the great toe when a large C is drawn around the outer malleolus at the ankle, the examiner again using the same noxious stimulus.

Numerous other signs, some of which follow, are important only as confirmatory signs and as indications of alteration in the disease process. Certainly a Babinski sign needs little confirmation. The same is not true of the other signs such as the Oppenheim (extension of the great toe on progressive distal pressure by the examiner's thumb on the tibia), the Gonda (extension of the great toe on forcible plantar flexion of the fourth toe), the Rossolimo (flexion of the toes on percussion of the ball of the foot), and the Bechterew (flexion of the toes on percussion of the dorsum of the foot). These other signs are of value only in giving some indication of the course of the disease. If a patient had a mildly present Babinski sign, and in the course of therapy or observation this has become more and more obvious and is now accompanied by confirmatory signs, then, of course, the patient's illness is progressing.

The various signs discussed fall into particular categories.

The signs indicative of corticospinal (pyramidal) tract involvement are weakness, spasticity, hyperactivity of the deep tendon reflexes, absence of abdominal reflexes, and the presence of Hoffmann's finger sign and Babinski's and Chaddock's toe signs. Those signs indicative of a "lower motor neuron" lesion are weakness, atrophy, areflexia, and hypotonia. If the lesion involves the neuron itself rather than the axon in the peripheral nerve, fasciculations also appear. The signs indicative of cerebellar involvement are intention tremor, dyssynergia, dysmetria, dysrhythmia, rebound phenomenon in the extremities, ataxia of gait, titubation (tremor on standing or walking), and scanning and slurring of speech.

SENSORY EXAMINATION

The usual modalities of sensation tested are vibratory, position, cutaneous pain, and light touch.

Vibratory sensation is tested with a 128-cycle tuning fork, since frequencies higher than this may not be well appreciated by some normal persons. It is important to note also that a normal decrease in vibratory sensation in the lower extremities occurs with increasing age. The proper observation of vibratory sense is begun by setting the tuning fork into active vibration and then touching it to the internal malleolus of one ankle. As soon as the patient acknowledges that he feels it, it is placed on the opposite side; then after he acknowledges it, it is again moved back and forth until vibratory sensation has disappeared bilaterally. It is thus possible to gauge the difference between the two sides. The vibratory sense can be tested in the same way over the iliac crests. When there is total absence in the lower extremities and at the iliac crest, the level may be identified in certain spinal cord lesions by testing over the individual spinous processes of the vertebrae. Vibratory sense in the upper extremities is tested in the same way as in the lower extremities.

Position sense is routinely investigated in the great toes and in the fingers by having the patient close his eyes before the digit to be examined is manually separated from all other digits. Touching the bedding or other objects is avoided to preclude the use of tactile cues. The toe or finger is then moved briskly in a vertical direction, and the patient is asked to tell whether it is up or down. In alert and highly cooperative patients it is better to move the digit slowly and have the patient indicate as soon as he is aware of movement. When done at the same rate of speed on the two sides, the evaluation of position sensation for purposes of comparison is sufficiently critical to show slight impairment on one side. Position sense in the great joints can be tested by having the patient point with the index finger to a particular digit. Then he closes his eyes, and again the entire extremity is put through the range of motion at the different joints, the patient following the digit with his own index finger. By this tracking procedure, impairment of position sense in the great joints can be determined.

Probably no part of the neurologic examination is more cumbersome and more fraught with errors, particularly for beginners, than the evaluation of **cutaneous pain sensation.** It is extremely important to avoid suggestion. Use of a leading question like ''Which one is sharper, this or this?'' obviously implies that one stimulus is expected to be sharper than the other and will lead the patient into errors. Comparison of pinprick sensation on the two sides of the face, both sides of the trunk, both upper extremities, and both lower extremities may be used to determine any difference between the two sides. Pinprick sensation is compared in a longitudinal axis of the patient for dermatomal or similar levels.

Closely allied to pain sensation is **temperature sensation.** Both modalities are carried in the lateral spinothalamic tract. Temperature sensation is not routinely tested but is additive to the demonstration of an area of analgesia. The patient is asked to indicate *hot* and *cold* as test tubes filled with ice and with hot water are touched to his skin. It is important that the examiner place the tubes in the same position on the patient's skin. If they are placed at different angles because one tube is held in the examiner's right hand and the other in the left hand, the patient will soon discern this difference.

The **light touch** sensation can be best tested by a small camel's-hair brush or wisp of cotton, and most patients can determine when either one or a few body hairs have been moved by a small whisk of the brush.

Stereognosis is tested by placing objects in the patient's hand while his eyes are closed or he is blindfolded and asking him to identify these objects by touch. Coins, marbles, pocketknives, and pens are good test objects. Cigarette lighters, for example, are not good because of the other clues that the patient may obtain from them: the click of the lid and the smell of fuel.

Special modalities, not routinely tested, include graphesthesia, or the ability to recognize numbers written on the skin. In carrying out this procedure, the numbers should always be written in such a way that if the patient's eyes were open, he would be in a position to read them. They should not be written at angles from his line of vision, even though his eyes are closed. The patient should first be apprised of what is going to happen; then a blunt object such as an orange stick or blunt end of a paper clip is placed on the skin, and the patient is asked, "Are you ready?" After he signals "yes," the writing of the figure is done slowly. Ironically, the numbers 1 and 7 (particularly 7) are extremely hard for patients to decipher.

Weight discrimination can be tested by placing a stack of coins on the supported hand. The patient is asked to compare one stack with another. Most patients can detect a difference that equals the weight of about 75 cents in quarters.

Texture discrimination can be tested at the bedside by using the fold of a sheet and the patient's robe or washcloth and asking him to distinguish between these as to thickness, softness, and other characteristics.

Two-point discrimination is determined by touching two points of a compass to the skin, measuring the range at which a patient can distinguish between one and two points. This distance varies from individual to individual and varies with different parts of the body. The distance at which two points can be distinguished is much less over the hand, greater over the arm, and much greater over the trunk. This is in accord with the amount of sensory cortex set aside for these regions.

Deep pain sensation is elicited by pressure exerted over a tendon, such as the Achilles tendon. It is necessary to avoid pinching the skin and confusing cutaneous with deep pain. Deep pain is therefore usually elicited by pressing the tendon (with the ball of the examiner's thumb) against the handle of the reflex hammer placed on the opposite side of the tendon.

Sensory extinction is tested by applying simultaneously to two sides of the body the same type of stimulus—pinprick or touch. In certain parietal lobe lesions the stimulus applied to the side opposite the lesion is perceived if it is the only stimulus but is masked and not appreciated when combined with a simultaneous stimulation on the normal side.

In all detailed sensory examinations it is important to take into consideration the patient's particular capabilities. A violinist, for example, has a most exquisite vibratory sense in his fingers; the expert typist or pianist will have excellent position sense in the fingers.

When the sensory examination is detailed, it can be extremely fatiguing for the patient, since so much concentration is required. It is often also fatiguing for the physician. And because it usually comes at the end of the detailed general physical and the rest of the neurologic examination, this adds to the element of fatigue. During the sensory examination it is best to allow the patient to open his eyes between the testing of the various modalities and to explain in this interval the nature of the next test. Also, when the sensory examination is important, it is best at the next examination, later in the day or the next day, to begin the entire neurologic examination with the study of the sensory functions.

CEREBRAL DOMINANCE

Cerebral dominance should be noted in the course of all neurologic examinations, particularly those with reference to cerebral disease. There are some clues to this in the course of the examination. Better developed musculature occurs in the dominant arm in tennis players, carpenters, and those engaged in other occupations or hobbies where much force is expended by one arm in contradistinction to the other.

Eyedness can be tested by giving the patient a card with a small hole punched in it and telling him to look through it at an object just an inch or so away from the hole in the paper. He will move it close and use the dominant eye. Another simple test is for the examiner to hold up two digits in a row and ask the patient to line them up in his vision. The eye with which he does this is his dominant eye.

Asking the patient to demonstrate in charade how he would thread a needle, drive a nail, put in a screw, or stir a pot on the stove determines **handedness.** The dominance is in the hand with the hammer or a stirring spoon, the hand that moves and carries out the motion in threading the needle—in general, the one that is active.

For testing **footedness** the patient is asked to stand on a chair, and the examiner notes which foot is placed on the chair to start the rise.

APHASIA

In the course of a careful neurologic examination, a reasonable preliminary assay of the language function is available in the patient's understanding of audible words and sounds, but more detailed examinations are necessary. Identification of objects by vision alone can well be carried out by the examiner's emptying his pockets of the usual coins, eyeglass or spectacle case, pen, notebook, lighter, and matches and then placing them in a battery in front of the patient and asking him to please pick up, for example, the cigarette lighter. This tests the auditory-verbal as well as the visual-object abilities. The reverse, pointing to the objects and asking the patient to name them, tests his word formulation abilities. He can be asked to identify actions shown in pantomime, such as brushing teeth, combing hair, tightening belt, or tying shoelaces.

The patient should be asked to write his own name. Only the severely aphasic will be unable to do this. The examinee is then instructed to write some simple phrase, such as "This is a nice day" or "This is the month of August." He is asked to draw a tree or a house to test his ability to recall objects from memory. He is given a proportionately simple drawing and asked to copy it. Then again he is asked to copy it, but this time the original and the first copy are covered. He may next be given a simple article in a newspaper to read aloud and decipher, or he may be shown a card on which is printed "please close your eyes" and told to do whatever is written on the card without reading it aloud. In this rather simple fashion the various modalities of language function can be tested.

EVALUATION OF MENTAL STATUS

Considerable information regarding the mental status is derived in the course of the history taking and examination. The physician should note whether the patient is oriented for time, place, and person. The state of the affect becomes obvious in the course of evaluation and indirectly by the patient's attitude toward his illness. The content of the patient's thoughts is also reasonably indicated. Paranoid trends or hallucinatory experiences should have been evolved if present in the course of questioning but can be specifically sought.

Of particular importance in neurology is the consideration of the organic-mental syndrome. This occurs with bilateral frontal lobe lesions of all types. This syndrome is characterized by a defective memory, especially regarding recent events, by impaired judgment, by difficulty in abstraction, by decreased arithmetic ability, and by alteration of affect.

Disturbances of consciousness occur in certain neurologic illnesses, varying from lethargy to deep coma. In the lethargic state the patient is not fully alert and tends to fall asleep. In the stuporous state the patient can be aroused only by vigorous stimulation. In coma the patient cannot be aroused. There are also comalike states due to lesions of the activating or reticular system, in which patients are awake or only lethargic, have little or no voluntary movement, have little or no potentiality for verbal communication. The eyes are open but without eye contact except in the locked-in syndrome due to a lesion transecting the upper pontine tegmentum.

CONCLUSION

In this outline of the neurologic examination, it is important to note that individual patients vary considerably in certain respects. Digital facility is excellent in persons whose occupations or hobbies necessitate it, for example, typists and pianists. These facilities may be very limited in persons with other occupations. In the examination patients should not be tested far beyond their limitations, especially in testing the language functions in aphasic patients. Due regard must be made for the patient's educational background. Giving someone with a relatively limited background a translation of "de Senectute" would be enough to invalidate the rest of the findings.

In detailing this emphasis on the neurologic examination, it was not intended to give the impression that the general physical examination is not important. The details of a good physical examination need not be described here. In every neurologic patient a careful general physicial examination is mandatory. The presence of masses in the breast, lymphadenopathy, or generalized wasting suggest a neoplastic disease. In patients with acute vascular accidents, the cardiac status, the presence of petechial hemorrhages in the conjunctivae or skin, and the presence of cardiac arrhythmias or dysrhythmias have obvious import. In patients with basal ganglia disease, the evidence of hepatic disease suggests a hepatic basal ganglia combination of disease. In the patient with cerebral aneurysm, pulsations over the posterior thoracic cage, hypertension in the upper extremities, and absent femoral pulses indicate the correlation of the aneurysm with coarctation of the aorta. Likewise, in patients with aneurysms the presence of a mass in the flank immediately suggests a coexistence of polycystic kidney disease.

Supernumerary nipples suggest the possibility of heredode-generative disease. Therefore clues derived from the general physical examination are equally important in arriving at the correct diagnosis and oftentimes are of even greater importance in the proper management of the patient's condition. However, since this book is concerned primarily with the nervous system, the detailed general examination is omitted—only from the descriptive aspects, not from the awareness of the physician!

REFERENCES

De Jong, R. N.: The neurologic examination, ed. 2, New York, 1958, Paul B. Hoeber, Inc., Medical Book Department of Harper & Row, Publishers, Inc.

Plum, F., and Posner, J.: Diagnosis of stupor and coma, Philadelphia, 1972, F. A. Davis Co.

Section on Neurology, Mayo Clinic: Clinical examination in neurology, ed. 4, Philadelphia, 1976, W. B. Saunders Co.

Strub, R. L., and Black, F. W.: The mental status examination in neurology, Philadelphia, 1977, F. A. Davis Co.

3 Clinical diagnostic tests

Various tests have been designed either to quantitate and augment the clinical observations of a particular function or to employ electric or other devices from other fields of science and bring their applications to the nervous system to assist in arriving at a diagnosis. In both cases the aim is to quantitate the information and pinpoint the diagnosis.

VISUAL FIELD STUDIES

The visual field studies are performed on a perimeter, a tangent screen, or a stereocampimeter. The usual perimeter suffices to give a reasonably accurate outline of the peripheral fields. On the tangent screen, however, the visual fields are studied with the patient at a distance of 1 meter from the black screen. White or colored objects of various sizes are brought into the patient's visual field.

The field is sufficiently large at a meter's distance that a reasonably accurate plotting of a scotoma can also be made. To accomplish this, the test object is placed in the center of the field and then is carried laterally in different parameters until the patient states that it is out of sight. If this occurs before the test object arrives at the previously determined peripheral margin of the field and if the object, progressing beyond this point, is again seen, a scotoma has been demonstrated. A normal blind spot in each eye is caused by the absence of retinal cells at the site of the nerve head itself. Two test objects are used in plotting peripheral fields. If the field defect is present with only one of the two test objects of different sizes, this is more likely to be caused by a focal retinal lesion than by an involvement of the nervous system pathways. If the visual pathways are involved, the defect is present regardless of the size of the object.

Tubular fields are rare in organic disease of the nervous system. These may occur in optic atrophy, particularly with a toxic basis. True tubular vision can be differentiated from the hysteric type by repeating the fields at different distances. If the size of the field is the same at 1 meter as at 5 meters, the basis is hysteria.

CALORIC TESTING

The caloric function of the vestibular apparatus can be easily tested at the bedside or in the office by injecting 3 ml of ice water into the ear of the patient who is recumbent in the supine position with the head elevated at about 30 degrees and turned to one side. The pinna is then held over the external auditory meatus. Nystagmus is tested for immediately. The nystagmus appears in about 20 seconds. There is slight past pointing, usually no nausea, and only slight subjective dizziness with a test done by this method. After the subsidence of the nystagmus, the opposite ear is tested in the same way. More detailed testing can be carried out, using larger amounts of cold or warm water and with the patient's head in different positions. From the neurologic standpoint, however, the physician is usually interested in knowing whether the vestibular apparatus is hypoactive, as in tumors of the eighth cranial nerve and in the late stages of Meniere's disease, or hyperactive, as in the early stages of Meniere's disease or labyrinthitis. Therefore, for neurologic purposes, definitive testing for each of the three canals is unnecessary.

Nystagmography is the documentation of the degree and duration of the nystagmus following a measured stimulus. This is accomplished by recording the eye movements by ink writer.

AUDIOMETRIC TESTING

Audiometric testing is done with a commercial apparatus that presents definitive sounds by means of one speaker to the ear undergoing tests and a masking noise to the ear not being tested. The definitive sounds are presented at various frequencies, and the patient indicates the point at which the sound disappears. With the position reversed and starting with an inaudible frequency, the patient indicates the point at which the sound is audible. These points are charted for both ears and indicate clearly the presence and type of hearing loss.

Special audiometric examinations, such as the Bekesy type, are of special value in the early diagnosis of lesions of the auditory branch of the eighth cranial nerve and especially in the diagnosis of acoustic neuromas. The Bekesy audiometry compares the observations on continuous and on interrupted tone presentations. The SISI test is the sharp increment sensitivity index. These tests together with tone decay and speech discrimination make it possible to diagnose or suspect acoustic neuromas before the appearance of gross neurologic signs, as when the neuroma is confined entirely to the internal auditory meatus.

CYSTOMETROGRAPHY

Cystometrography is the study of urinary bladder function. It is accomplished by injecting sterile fluid into the bladder, measuring the bladder tone and the amount of fluid the bladder will hold, and determining the presence of emptying contractions. This is usually done by dripping fluid slowly into a catheter, having a manometric device cut into the mechanism so that the pressure can be observed and/or recorded.

The bladder tone rises rather slowly as the fluid gathers in the bladder. Small contractions of the bladder appear at a capacity of 50 to 100 ml. The normal bladder can hold 300 ml without too much difficulty. Then emptying contractions appear, and the patient is well aware of fullness of the bladder. In the hypotonic or atonic bladder, 500 ml or more can be run into the bladder with a slight rise in bladder pressure, with no emptying contractions, and without the patient's awareness that the bladder is full. In the hypertonic bladder, pressure rises rapidly, and with only 25 or 50 ml of capacity emptying contractions may appear. This may even be the total amount of urine that the bladder will contain. Simple catheterization may reveal the presence of significant residual urine. This is also an indication of bladder dysfunction.

The tests for bladder function are important in diagnosing suspected cord disease, when neurologic findings are not definitive. Cystometric evaluation of the bladder is helpful also in studying patients with significant mental changes who soil themselves, and the question arises whether this is on a neurologic basis or is merely a reflection of the mental status. When the apparent incontinence is due to the impaired mental status, the cystometrogram is normal.

ELECTROENCEPHALOGRAPHY

Electroencephalography is most useful in the study of epilepsy, quite useful in the localization of cerebral lesions (particularly those close to the cortex), and valuable in the study of metabolic disorders such as hepatic coma and in determining cerebral death. This test is essentially the recording of the electrical activity of the brain. The recording is usually done on paper by ink writers. Multiple areas of the brain must be recorded simultaneously, and considerable sophistication is necessary in interpreting the tracings. This is a complex field in itself.

In epilepsy, electroencephalography is invaluable. This test aids in confirming the presence of epilepsy in doubtful cases, aids in determining whether the seizures originate from a particular focus of the brain, and gives some help in differentiating the minor seizure types (as psychomotor from petit mal). In the management of the patient's condition, the value other than for these facts is limited. The patient is treated, not his brain waves. Therefore dosage levels and duration of medications are not contingent on the electroencephalographic findings. The brain wave patterns are helpful in advising epileptic parents regarding the possibilities of producing epileptic offspring, particularly when both parents are studied.

In addition to electroencephalographic recording from scalp electrodes, recordings can be made from deeper structures. The simplest ways of doing this are to employ electrodes placed in the nasopharynx or needle-inserted electrodes under the maxilla and touching the sphenoid bone. Recordings can be obtained from the base of the frontal and mesial aspects of the temporal lobes using this technique. Nasopharyngeal electrodes may cross, however, and it is important if a unilateral discharge occurs that the electrode placement by ascertained accurately by use of an x-ray film.

STUDY OF EVOKED POTENTIALS

In electroencephalography the administration of a stimulus does not apparently alter the record. For example, if a light flash is presented, no change can be seen in records from the occipital lobe of the normal individual. The response is masked by the usual electrical activity. If, however, repeated stimuli are administered and the record is analyzed by computer, the response is evident. In disease processes the response may be delayed, abnormal, or absent. This process then can indicate lesions in certain parts of the nervous system because the appropriate pathways are altered.

The alteration of the visually evoked responses is of value in the demonstration of subclinical involvement of the optic pathways and is of special value in the diagnosis of multiple sclerosis. The test for this purpose is often referred to as VECA or VER.

The administration of auditory stimuli and the study of the responses are of value in determining lesions interfering with the auditory pathways. These pathways are both diverse and diffuse, and therefore localization of brain stem lesions by this technique is of value.

ELECTROMYOGRAPHY

In its broadest interpretation, electromyography includes not only the recording of the electrical activity of the muscles themselves but also studies of the electrical responses of the peripheral nerves. The recording of muscle activity may indicate denervation by the presence of fibrillations or anterior horn cell disease by the presence of fasciculations. Less gross changes than these include alterations of the phasic potentials of the muscles. It is customary to listen to the discharges as amplified as well as to record them.

An expert electromyographer can often distinguish polymyositis from other myopathies. Electromyography is necessary to distinguish myasthenia gravis from the other myasthenic-like syndromes, for example, the Eaton-Lambert syndrome. With tetanic stimulation there is a progressive decrement in muscle response in true myasthenia, whereas in other conditions after a period of decrement that is a terminal increase in response. In myotonia the discharges elicited by a minor stimulus such as moving the needle slightly are repetitive and prolonged and sound like a "dive bomber." The characteristics of myasthenia and of myotonia can be elicited even when the usual clinical responses are absent or equivocal.

When the lesion occurs in a peripheral nerve, it is possible in many instances to document the level of the lesion by the demonstration of impairment of nerve conduction. An electrical stimulus is administered to a peripheral nerve, and the electrical activity of the innervated muscle is recorded. The time between administration and arrival of stimulus at the muscle can be recorded, and interference with transmission can thus be determined.

ROUTINE RADIOGRAPHY

In routine films of the skull, the lateral anteroposterior and posteroanterior views should be routinely scrutinized in an orderly fashion. First, the facial bones are noted for any obvious fracture. Second, the contents of the various sinuses are observed for evidence of sinusitis and for the presence of neoplasms within the sinuses. Third, the outer and inner tables are followed carefully for any evidence of fracture or erosion.

Fourth, the sella is observed for its size and the degree of calcification of the clinoids. The same procedure is followed in the anteroposterior and posteroanterior views. If the radiograph is taken from the brow to the base of the skull, the outline of the internal auditory meatus is noted.

Fractures are indicated by lines in the bones of the skull. Certain fractures, notably those involving only the base of the skull (particularly the cribriform plate), are difficult if not impossible to visualize. Fractures of the calvarium may be depressed. Occasionally, when tabs of meninges are caught within the fracture line, the fracture line widens progressively over a long period of time.

Increased intracranial pressure is indicated by beaten silver markings in the skull (although not necessarily abnormal in children under the age of 14 years), by decalcification of the sella and clinoids, and in young children by separation of suture lines.

Normal calcifications occur in the skull as follows: in the pineal body, in the habenular region, in the glomus of the choroid plexus, and in the falx. Displacement of the calcifications may indicate a space-taking lesion or an atrophic lesion. Care must be taken in interpreting asymmetric positioning of the calcified glomi of the choroid plexus, since the calcification may not be in the same position within each lateral ventricle and thus may give rise to an appearance of ventricular distortion.

In pituitary neoplasms, particularly chromophobic and eosinophilic adenomas, the **sella** is **enlarged** and ballooned, and the clinoids may be displaced upward.

Erosion of the bone occurs in metastatic tumors such as carcinomas and multiple myelomas. These are multiple bilateral destructive lesions and, depending on the nature of the metastasizing tumor, may have some osteoblastic activity about them. Meningiomas may present an erosion of the bone with the development of new bone beyond the erosion and a peculiar radial-like spicule formation in the new bone and in the area of bony destruction. Osteomas appears as well-demonstrated, opaque lesions within the bone. Epidermoids are rare tumors of the skull with clear and highly translucent, well-demarcated, almost geographic erosions of bone, and with very little osteo-blastic activity around the edges.

Abnormal calcifications may occur in blood vessels. These are most evident in the carotid arteries and are seen in the area of the sella. Occasionally calcifications occur in neoplasms, particularly in the less malignant primary neoplasms such as meningiomas, oligodendrogliomas, and astrocytomas.

TOMOGRAPHY

Tomography permits a "slice" view of the skull in a pre-determined plane, thus eliminating overlying and underlying structures from being visualized. This is especially useful for studies at the base of the skull, for example, the internal audi-tory meati or when the condition of the sella is in doubt.

Computerized tomography

Computerized tomography of the brain is the most sig-nificant advance in the technology of neurologic diagnosis in the last fifty years. This consists of the computerized summa-tion of multiple x-rays of the head taken at specific levels and is known as EMI (for Electronic Musical Instrument—the manufacturer of the first such apparatus) or as CT or CAT scan (for computerized axial tomography). This procedure requires the careful placing of the patient's head in the instrument for about 40 minutes. Thousands of x-ray studies are gathered, placed on tape, analyzed by computer, and printed out. The printouts show at a number of almost horizontal levels or "slices" the bony structures, cortex, ventricles, larger cis-terns, calcifications, and changes in brain tissue density due to lesions. Alterations in density can be further delineated by the intravenous injection of contrast material.

DOPPLER STUDIES

The Doppler effect can be employed for the noninvasive study of extracranial blood vessels and their blood flow. Ultrasonic impulses are presented methodically along the course of a vessel wall, and the reflected return is recorded. The circulating red blood cells are the reflecting agent. By this means the rate of, absence of, and direction of flow can be determined.

CONTRAST RADIOGRAPHY

Contrast studies are often necessary to localize neoplasms and other intracranial and intraspinal lesions. The replacement of cerebrospinal fluid by air permits radiographic visualization of the ventricular system, and when the air is introduced by way of lumbar puncture **(pneumoencephalography),** the arachnoid cisterns fill as well. Lumbar pneumoencephalography is employed in patients suspected of having atrophic lesions and in patients who might have neoplasms but do not have papilledema and are not suspected of having posterior fossa tumors.

Ventriculography is a surgical procedure with the direct replacement of ventricular fluid by air, accomplished by means of one or more burr or small drill holes placed in the skull and by puncture of the ventricles with a special needle. Whether the lesion is atrophic or a mass, the air studies indicate the location of the lesion by alteration in size, shape, or position of ventricular, subarachnoid, or cisternal spaces.

Angiography is the injection of radiopaque dye into the carotid or vertebral artery and the rapid visualization in a series of x-ray films of the passage of the dye through the cerebral vascular system. Intra-arterial catheterization, using either the brachial or femoral artery for the route of entrance, has become more popular and in capable hands leads to complete visualization of the major vessels and their branches, offering a completeness of study. This is especially valuable in the study of cerebrovascular lesions and is necessary in evaluating for vascular reconstructive surgery in the neck. This procedure is of value in demonstrating (1) the presence of occlusion of major vessels, (2) the presence of aneurysms, (3) displacement of vessels, indicating the presence of a mass, and (4) possibly the type of tumor. A meningioma, for example, often appears well outlined and well defined. Glioblastoma multiforme, on the other hand, is less well defined in outline but presents a faint tumorlike blush appearing deep in the brain tissue. Venous sinus thrombosis may also be demonstrated by this technique. In infants whose sagittal sinuses are suspected of being occluded, a **sinogram** can be carried out by the injection of dye directly into the superior sagittal sinus at the anterior fontanel.

RADIOISOTOPIC SCANNING

Radioisotopic scanning consists of an intravenous injection of an appropriate isotope followed at the proper time interval by Geiger counter scanning of the cranial surface. The isotopic agents used are albumin tagged with radioactive iodine (RISA), Technetium-99, and radioactive mercury. The latter is used in cases in which lesions are suspected in the posterior fossa or the temporal regions. Since, in a RISA scan, the muscles over these regions also pick up the isotope, scanning is more difficult with serum albumin. Technetium-99 is more widely used. This preparation has many of the advantages of radioactive mercury, and in addition the scan can be performed in a shorter time. Technetium brain scanning also permits some determination of blood flow in the great vessels in the neck.

Neoplasms are frequently revealed by the scanning technique. Large areas of encephalomalacia will also accumulate the isotope, and areas of increased blood supply, such as occurs in hemangiomas, will also be evidenced.

Radioactive scanning can also be performed after the intrathecal injection of the isotope, with some value for scanning of the spinal canal, but its greatest value is in the diagnosis of occult hydrocephalus. Serial scanning over a 24- to 48-hour period after injection may reveal a backflow of cerebrospinal fluid into a dilated ventricular system and the absence of isotope over the cortex.

Emission tomography which combines the techniques of isotope scanning and computerized tomography, is under investigation at the present time. By the appropriate selection of isotopes, this should lead to the possibility of studying biochemical changes in the brain. This holds considerable promise for the future, especially in the area of metabolic disorders.

MYELOGRAPHY

Myelography is the radiographic study of the spinal canal by means of a contrast substance (usually Pantopaque) injected by way of lumbar puncture. The dye is removed at the completion of the test.

The column of dye is observed fluoroscopically with the patient on a tilt table, and pertinent films are taken. Obstructions to the flow are evident, and the level of the lesion is determined. Indeed, the nature of the lesion is obvious, at least as to differentiation between intramedullary and extramedullary masses. It is important to study the entire spinal cord during myelography and to record the uppermost level observed fluoroscopically if this is not documented by film.

CEREBROSPINAL FLUID STUDIES

Cerebrospinal fluid is almost invariably obtained by lumbar puncture and rarely, at present, by cisternal puncture. The lumbar puncture should be performed with the patient recumbent on his side. Local anesthesia is employed. The needle is inserted in an interspace between the second lumbar and the first sacral vertebrae. The **choice of interspace** depends to some extent on the diagnosis being considered. For example, in a patient with a cerebrovascular accident, the choice of interspace is inconsequential. However, in the patient suspected of having a ruptured intervertebral disk at the third to fourth lumbar interspace, the puncture should be performed below that level to obtain the maximum number of abnormalities in the fluid. The site of every lumbar puncture should always be recorded in the chart for future reference.

The **pressure** is carefully recorded by water manometer. A pressure over 200 mm H_2O is considered abnormal. If the pressure is somewhat above this, the knees should be drawn down from the abdomen and the patient should be asked to take several deep breaths and reassured that the procedure is virtually over and there will be no further pain. In this manner the pressure, if actually normal, is brought within the normal range.

Manometrics (Queckenstedt test) can be determined by the occlusion of the jugular veins. Normally, within 10 seconds after the jugular veins have been occluded, either manually or by a blood pressure cuff about the neck at a pressure of 20 mm Hg, the cerebrospinal fluid pressure increases from 150 to 400 mm H_2O and promptly drops back within 10 seconds after the release of pressure. A control test for this is conducted by pressing on the abdomen, which raises the pressure in the same period of time to about 250 mm H_2O. If no rise occurs on either jugular or abdominal compression, the bevel of the needle is obstructed by tabs of arachnoid or by a nerve root, and the failure to rise on jugular compression is of no significance. If intracranial problems are suspected, the maneuver will not be definitive and may seriously affect the patient's status. Therefore this maneuver should be performed only in patients suspected by having a block in the spinal subarachnoid space. A complete myelogram is much more informative and in practice has almost outmoded the study of spinal fluid dynamics.

The first few drops of spinal fluid are employed for cell count; the next 5 ml are sent to the laboratory for chemical determination, then 5 ml are drawn for serologic testing and 5 ml for gamma globulin determination or colloidal gold determination. It is always wise to draw an extra 5 ml (unless contraindicated) in case the laboratory results are doubtful or the fluid is inadvertently lost. The closing pressure is noted.

The **color** of the fluid is observed for the presence of blood or xanthochromic discoloration. **Cells** should be counted immediately. Normally there are not more than three to five lymphocytes per cubic millimeter; five is the highest number considered to be normal. There may be as many as 200 red blood cells in a normal lumbar puncture. These are not crenated and are due to the procedure. They are found when the cell count is performed on the first few drops of fluid. The cell count may reveal not only an abnormality in the number of cells but also the presence of abnormal (such as malignant) cells. Rarely even gitter cells may be seen in the fluid of a patient with a massive encephalomalacia. Torula can be identified by the house officer counting the cells, and occasionally even such rare entities as trichinae are noted by the intern or resident.

Normal **protein content** of the spinal fluid varies from 15 to 45 mg/100 ml; a total protein content of over 50 mg/100 ml is abnormal. Spinal fluids with protein contents over 1,500 mg/100 ml clot at room temperature.

The spinal fluid **sugar** content should be measured quantitatively when there is an increase in cells, since it is helpful only in determining the severity of meningitis and to some extent in differentiating the type of meningitis (for example, benign lymphocytic meningitis from tuberculous meningitis). The spinal fluid sugar content is also decreased by the presence of malignant cells such as carcinomatous or sarcomatous cells in the spinal fluid.

The chloride content of the spinal fluid is seldom measured nowadays, since it is of no aid in diagnosis.

The **colloidal gold test** is still employed in some laboratories but has largely been replaced by **gamma globulin determinations.** The gamma globulin content is important in its relationship to the total protein content; that is, the significant figure is the percentage of the spinal fluid protein that is composed of gamma globulin. When this percentage is over 20%, it is definitely abnormal, occurring in patients with multiple sclerosis, neurosyphilis, and illnesses that produce elevations and abnormalities of serum globulins.

Various **serologic tests** are employed, such as the complement fixation tests, the *Treponema pallidum* immune adherence (TPIA), and the *Treponema* immobilization test (TPI), in that order. If a complement fixation positive result is suspected of being false, the TPIA is employed. The TPI is the most accurate test but is difficult and expensive.

Traumatic tap vs. subarachnoid hemorrhage

When blood appears in the spinal fluid at the time of the lumbar puncture, the physician performing the tap can usually differentiate between a bloody tap and a true subarachnoid hemorrhage. In a traumatic puncture the fluid may clot; this does not occur in a subarachnoid hemorrhage. Also in the traumatic tap, if the fluid in the needle does not clot, it becomes progressively clearer. Both the red and white cells should be counted, even though the tap is traumatic. A reasonable approximation of white cell count of the bloody spinal fluid can be determined by using the formula R.B.C. (blood): W.B.C.(blood) = R.B.C.(CSF):x, where x is the suspected number of white blood cells in the spinal fluid. If the actual cell count is much greater than the expected count, it suggests that the patient had an increase in white cell count in the spinal fluid before the bloody tap. Also, the total protein content evaluation may be corrected by computing 1 mg of protein per 1,000 red blood cells present in the spinal fluid. Although the puncture is traumatic, some immediate results can be obtained from the fluid.

The various diagnostic procedures offer a wide selection to the physician. Most of them are costly, some of them are painful, and a few carry significant morbidity factors. The choice of procedure therefore must be rational and logical. Moreover, procedures that are potentially dangerous or painful should not be undertaken if the physician will not proceed with the findings. For example, an angiogram is not indicated in a patient who may have cerebrovascular disease but whose general medical condition precludes any possibility of reconstructive vascular surgery.

REFERENCES

Ambrose, J.: Computerized transverse axial scanning (tomography). II. Clinical applications, Br. J. Radiol. **46:**1023, 1973.

Blackwell, E., Merory, J., Toole, J. F., and McKinney, W.: Doppler ultrasound scanning of the carotid bifurcation, Arch. Neurol. **34:**145, 1977.

Cohen, H. L., and Brumlik, J.: Manual of electroneuromyography, New York, 1976, Harper & Row, Publishers, Inc.

Davidoff, L. M., and Epstein, B. S.: The abnormal pneumoencephalogram, ed. 2, Springfield, Ill., 1955, Charles C Thomas, Publisher.

Ecker, A., and Reimschneider, P. A.: Angiographic localization of intracranial nerves, Springfield, Ill., 1955, Charles C Thomas, Publisher.

Fishman, R. A.: Cerebrospinal fluid. In Baker, A. B., editor: Clinical neurology, ed. 3, New York, 1975, Harper & Row, Publishers, Inc.

Harrington, D. O.: The visual fields: a textbook and atlas of clinical perimetry, ed. 3, St. Louis, 1971, The C. V. Mosby Co.

Kiloh, L. G., McComas, A. J., and Osselton, J. W.: Clinical electroencephalography, ed. 3, London, 1972, Butterworth & Co.

Merritt, H. H., and Fremont-Smith, F.: The cerebrospinal fluid, Philadelphia, 1938, W. B. Saunders Co.

Newton, T. H., and Potts, D. G.: Radiology of the skull and brain, vol. I. The skull, 1971; vol. II. Angiography, 1974; vol. III. Anatomy and pathology, 1977, St. Louis, The C. V. Mosby Co.

Pendergass, E. P., Schweffer, J. P., and Holles, P. J.: The head and neck in roentgen diagnosis, ed. 2, Springfield, Ill., 1956, Charles C Thomas, Publisher.

Ramsey, R. G.: Computed tomography of the brain; advanced exercises in diagnostic radiology, vol. 9, Philadelphia, 1977, W. B. Saunders Co.

Section on Neurology, Mayo Clinic: Clinical examinations in neurology, ed. 4, Philadelphia, 1976, W. B. Saunders Co.

Smorto, M. P., and Basmajian, J. V.: Electrodiagnosis; a handbook for neurologists, New York, 1977, Harper & Row, Publishers, Inc.

Wood, E. H.: An atlas of myelography. Prepared for the Registry of Radiology in Pathology, Washington, D. C., 1948, Registry Press.

PART TWO   **CLINICAL NEUROLOGIC ENTITIES**

4 Vascular diseases

Cerebrovascular disease is the third most important cause of death in the United States and is responsible for an even greater morbidity. In general, cerebral hemorrhage is more frequently responsible for deaths and encephalomalacia is responsible for chronic morbidity.

ENCEPHALOMALACIAS

Under the term "encephalomalacia" are grouped those entities whose etiology is due to inadequate blood flow to a part of the brain, resulting in softening of the deprived brain tissue. The maintenance of an adequate blood supply is contingent on many factors. Impairment of cerebral blood flow may be the result of changes in the cerebral blood vessels, the characteristics of the circulating blood, or of the general circulation. The changes in the cerebral vessels may be stenotic, on the basis of arteriosclerosis with a resultant narrowing of the lumen or may be due to thrombosis, vasculitis, or the lodging of an embolus. Changes in the circulating blood include alterations of cells (as sickling) in cellular content or number (as in anemia and polycythemia) or in the levels of those constituents essential to cerebral metabolism, oxygen, and glucose. Changes in the general circulation that critically reduce blood pressure and blood flow include myocardial infarction and the various shock states. Combinations of these factors may lead to a relative insufficiency. When the lumen of the vessel has been considerably encroached on by the presence of atheromatous plaques and when, for some other reasons, cerebral blood flow is decreased, a critical point for nutrition of the brain tissue occurs.

47

If this critical state of oxygenation and glucose supply is maintained for 10 minutes, the involved brain tissue will die. The importance of relative insufficiency has long been recognized. Patients with myocardial insufficiency may present with the clinical picture of cerebrovascular accident, and the prompt treatment of the cardiac condition may result in the prompt remission of the neurologic symptoms.

Actual thrombosis of a vessel can be demonstrated in about one third of the cases of encephalomalacia. Emboli are not common as a cause of encephalomalacia but, when they do occur, may arise from intramural thrombi in the heart or may be paradoxical and arise from varicosities or, indeed, any other emboli. Emboli also arise from ulcerated plaques and from thrombi in the cerebral vasculature. Vasculitis, or inflammatory disease of the vessel wall, in former years was most commonly syphilitic. With the decrease in neurosyphilis and, indeed, syphilis itself, this has become uncommon. However, the group of collagenous diseases, particularly polyarteritis nodosa and lupus erythematosus, produce encephalomalacia syndromes by affecting the cerebral vessels. Usually this does not occur until after evidence of the collagenous disease in other tissues, such as skin, renal tissue, and others, but there are rare instances when the presenting symptoms are caused by involvement of the cerebral circulation.

The **pathology** of the brain lesions is the same regardless of which of these factors has caused the decrease in blood flow. In the first several hours loss of nerve cells and edema occurs, with beginning proliferation of microglia. Lysis of the tissue occurs on about the third day, with caseous necrosis in infarcts of any appreciable size. Then begins an astrocytic walling off of the broken-down tissue. If the lesion is of any appreciable size, a cyst is formed.

Clinically, patients with encephalomalacia due to thrombosis, stenosis, or relative insufficiency are usually over the age of 50 years, have had some history of hypertension, and often have cardiovascular renal disease. The patients may have had prodromas of headaches and even transient focal neurologic symptoms. Usually the onset is acute, often occurring at a period of decreased activity, for example, while the patient is asleep during the night. The maximal damage is generally present immediately or shortly thereafter. However, this is not necessarily true, since thrombi may propagate and extend along a vessel involving more and more branches so that the neurologic symptomatology may increase over a period of days.

The nature of the symptomatology, of course, depends on the brain area involved. Paralysis or paresis of one side of the body occurs when the motor cortex or the corticospinal projection is involved. At the onset the paralyzed parts are flaccid with decreased tendon reflexes, but gradually an increased tone or spasticity occurs attended by hyperactive tendon reflexes and the classic plantar signs. The spasticity is extensor in the lower extremities and flexor in the upper extremities, thus emphasizing the antigravity nature of the tonus. The motor weakness is greatest distally, that is, in those parts with the most liberal cerebral cortical representation.

When the lesion is in the dominant hemisphere, language functions are disturbed and the patient has an aphasia. The nature of the aphasia depends, of course, on the location of the lesion and possibly to a considerable extent on the patient's own learning mechanisms. Aphasia may be expressive and predominantly in the motor sphere. The patient then has full understanding of concepts and the appropriate words but is unable to verbalize. In amnestic aphasia the concepts are retained and the words are lost. This may be described as a loss of the dictionary. In receptive, or auditory-verbal, aphasia the patient is unable to comprehend the spoken word.

Visual field defects, particularly hemianopia, occur in lesions of the occipital and temporal regions. For this to be the sole presenting symptom is rather unusual. Rarely this may present as a reading difficulty, particularly when there is a hemianopia in the left fields.

Sensory changes are almost complete when the sensory pathways to the posterolateral ventral nuclei of the thalamus are involved. When the disruption is between these relay nuclei and the sensory cortex or of the sensory cortex alone, sensory deficits are less severe insofar as recognition of pain is concerned, but cortical sensory functions (weight and texture discrimination, two-point discrimination, and stereognosis) are impaired. When the posterior lobules are involved, agnostic sensibilities are impaired. When the lesion is in the inferior parietal lobule of the dominant hemisphere, Gerstmann's syndrome (acalculia, agraphia, finger agnosia, and confusion of laterality) occurs. If the lesion is in the inferior parietal lobule of the minor hemisphere, the syndrome of anosognosia occurs with the denial of the left hemiplegia and even of the left side of the body. When a vascular lesion due to occlusion of the thalamogeniculate artery involves the posterolateral ventral nucleus of the thalamus, the patient may have complete anesthesia on the opposite side of the body, which is a peculiar, painful anesthesia with severe intractable pain produced by the slightest touch (anesthesia dolorosa).

Some vascular lesions can be rather sharply localized. In recent times and with the use of arteriography, it has become evident that the old criteria for the strict localization of lesions as to which vessel is involved are less accurate than was formerly supposed. In this regard it is noteworthy that complete occlusion of the internal carotid artery often presents a clinical picture of occlusion of the middle cerebral artery. Indeed, in autopsy studies of carotid artery occlusion, the maximum damage to the brain is in the distribution of the middle cerebral artery.

When vascular neurosyphilis was prevalent, many syndromes of the brain stem were recorded and characterized by alternating paralysis. Many of these were due to involvement of a branch of the basilar artery, which destroyed the corticospinal tract and one or more cranial nerves on the same side, thus giving cranial nerve signs on the same side and paralysis of the extremities on the other (for example, the paralysis of the sixth cranial nerve on the right side with paralysis of the left arm and leg). These syndromes are rarely seen now, since neurosyphilis is so rare.

One of the brain stem syndromes, however, that is usually caused by arteriosclerosis is still common and is a well-defined syndrome. This is the lateral medullary syndrome or the syndrome of the posteroinferior cerebellar artery. The symptomatology is due to brain stem involvement rather than to partial destruction of the cerebellum, since this artery also supplies part of the brain stem. This syndrome in its pure state consists of sudden onset of vertigo, ataxia, and, on the side of the lesion, Horner's syndrome, paralysis of the vocal cord and perhaps the palate, anesthesia of the face, and a contralateral analgesia of the trunk and extremities.

The syndrome of basilar artery occlusion is important. This is characterized by disturbances of consciousness, bilateral cranial nerve involvement from the third to the twelfth cranial nerve, with impairment of extraocular movements, often with diplopia, involvement of speech, swallowing, and bilateral pyramidal tract signs.

Transient ischemic attacks (TIAs) are temporary episodes of focal cerebral dysfunction of vascular origin. The onset is acute, usually in less than 2 minutes. The symptoms last for only a few minutes and rarely as long as a day; they clear as rapidly as they occurred. The symptomatology may be that of either the carotid or basivertebral systems.

Many patients with completed strokes give histories of having had TIAs. However, adequate prospective studies of patients with TIAs are not yet available to provide the incidence of the development of completed strokes in these patients. Studies which are available suggest that a range of 10% to 32% of patients will develop strokes.

In the laboratory studies, routine radiographic study of the skull is occasionally helpful in demonstrating existing calcification in the cerebral vessels. If the cerebral lesion is large, the calcified pineal body may be displaced by the edema of the hemisphere. This is most likely to occur if the patient is comatose.

Cerebrospinal fluid studies are of value in differentiating between cerebral hemorrhage and encephalomalacia, since the spinal fluid is normal in 80% of patients with cerebral thrombosis and is bloody with increased intracranial pressure in 80% of patients with cerebral hemorrhage.

Arteriography plays an important role in the diagnosis of the presence of encephalomalacia and may demonstrate an occluded vessel or a plaque of sufficient size to impair circulation. There is, of course, some hazard (particularly in the older patient) in carrying out arteriography. When adequate definition of the disease process is necessary for institution of therapy, arteriography is essential and justified.

Nonhazardous laboratory tests that can be performed on the patient with a cerebrovascular accident include ophthalmodynamometry. The ocular pressure so measured is usually about two thirds of the systolic and one half of the diastolic pressures as measured brachially. A significant decrease in ocular values on the side opposite the clinical signs indicates occlusion of the carotid artery below the takeoff of the ophthalmic artery. Careful ophthalmoscopic examination with the pupils dilated may show the presence of emboli, either cholesterol from an ulcerated plaque or thrombotic in nature.

Noninvasive techniques aimed at the study of the great vessels in the neck include soft tissue x-ray films of the neck to demonstrate vascular calcification and blood flow studies, using either the Doppler effect or the scanning of an isotope flow.

For the study of the intracranial contents, EMI or CT scanning may not show the encephalomacic lesion for the first several days after the stroke. However, a hemorrhage of appreciable size will be evident immediately, so the CT scan is of immediate value in the differential diagnosis.

Radioisotopic scanning, particularly with the newer technetium-99 preparation, in a short period of time may be used to indicate the location of the lesion. This technique also holds promise of prognostic significance and, like CT scans, may be used to indicate the limitation of the lesion as well. Echoencephalography may be employed as an indicator of shift of the intracranial contents, either due to massive intracerebral hemorrhage or to edema.

The **general or supportive treatment** of the stroke patient is contingent on the patient's general condition. Many patients with encephalomalacia are not rendered unconscious. However, the comatose patient requires attention to life preservation factors such as aeration, nutrition, fluids, and electrolytes. Adequate oxygenation is obviously necessary, and posturing the patient for proper aeration is **important.** Airways may be necessary. It is important to collect the urine to prevent the development of decubiti. Condom drainage is best for the male patient. Indwelling catheterization is usually necessary for women. Convulsive seizures can occur during the acute phase of a stroke and can be controlled by intravenous administration of diazepam or sodium phenobarbital. Chlorpromazine can be administered for restlessness and/or nausea and vomiting. If severe hypertension (systolic pressure above 200 mm Hg) is present, antihypertensive therapy is indicated to lower the pressure to about 160 mm Hg.

In most instances of encephalomalacia there is no acute problem in the **supportive treatment.** Sometimes, however, because of the cerebral edema and distortion and compression of brain stem vessels, herniation may develop and cause perivascular hemorrhages in the brain stem. This is indicated by further disturbances of consciousness, nuchal rigidity without a Kernig's sign, development of bilateral pyramidal tract signs, hiccoughs, and respiratory irregularities. It is necessary to treat these patients vigorously to reduce their increased intracranial pressure. This can best be accomplished by repeated injections of mannitol or 50 ml of 50% glucose or by the use of magnesium sulfate enemas. Urea solutions can be injected intravenously if there is no possibility of concomitant hemorrhage. The **specific treatment** of encephalomalacia is concerned with the return of an adequate blood flow to the part. Ideally this should be accomplished within 10 minutes of the ictus, since this is the period of time in which the nerve cells begin to die. The measures aimed at return of adequate blood flow may be surgical or medical.

Medical methods include employing cerebral vasodilating agents and anticoagulants. The best known cerebral vasodilator at present is carbon dioxide in 5% mixture with 95% oxygen, which can be administered through a mask for 15-minute periods each hour for the first 48 hours. It is unlikely that after this time it will accomplish anything. There is some indication, however, that by increasing general cerebral blood flow, vasodilators may, in fact, shunt blood away from the ischemic zone.

Anticoagulant therapy is of value only in the treatment of thrombin emboli and of the evolving stroke. When a stroke is completed, there is no evidence of any value being derived from anticoagulant therapy. However, even in the patient with an evolving stroke, anticoagulant therapy is contraindicated if hypertension or bleeding tendencies are present. Heparin is frequently employed in the acute phase of anticoagulation, but in the long-term handling of the patient coumarin preparations are preferable. The condition of patients who are receiving anticoagulation therapy must be observed carefully in regard to their clotting or partial thromboplastin times. The role of thrombolytic agents is not yet clarified. Daily administrations of acetylsalicylic acid appear to have some effect in preventing further episodes in patients with transient ischemic attacks.

Surgical procedures have opened a new area in the management of occlusive cerebrovascular disease. By extending angiography to include the vessels as they arise from the arch of the aorta, in some of the cases of intermittent syndromes of the carotid artery, plaques are found at the origin or at the bifurcation of the common carotid artery. At present a number of surgical procedures are being performed in this type of patient and in those whose arteries have been completely occluded. Critical evaluation of these results is yet awaited. However, at this time it appears that the best surgical results are obtained in patients with little or no evidence of permanent neurologic deficit, whose occlusive disease involves only one of the major vessels and the obstruction involves at least 80% of the lumen.

The developing field of microsurgery also holds promise. By operating under microscopic control, it is possible to perform anastomoses of the more superficial cerebral vessels with extra cranial vessels, for example, the middle cerebral artery with the temporal artery.

In the treatment of encephalomalacia due to emboli, it is important that the source of the emboli be found and controlled, for example, by high saphenous vein ligation for varicosities in the lower extremities and the proper control of cardiac dysrhythmia. Anticoagulation therapy is indicated in the treatment of patients with emboli, especially when these are due to mitral stenosis and atrial fibrillation. Such treatment reduces the incidence of recurrent emboli. In the patient with encephalomalacia due to vasculitis caused by collagenous disease, the proper and appropriate steroid therapy for the disease entity is indicated.

DURAL VENOUS SINUS THROMBOSIS

Thromobisis of the dural venous sinuses occurs primarily in childhood, unless it is associated with infection of structures contiguous to the sinuses. The most common of the sinus thromboses occurred in the lateral sinus and was associated with mastoiditis. The next most common was cavernous sinus thrombosis secondary to facial infections, but with the better control of infections, these have become uncommon. In infants and young children sinus thrombosis occurred in relation to disturbances of fluid balance and hemoconcentration, such as with burns or long-standing diarrhea. The syndrome may also be due to a blood dyscrasia such as spherocytic or sickle cell dysmorphism of the erythrocytes. The problem is basically an occlusion of a sinus with damming back of blood into the vessels of the drained area, destruction of capillaries, and perivascular hemorrhage and softening of the brain tissue.

The **clinical signs** depend on the sinus involved in the thrombotic process. When the superior sagittal sinus is occluded, the cerebral cortex is involved with resultant motor and sensory deficits and seizures. When the vein of Galen is occluded, the basal ganglia are involved with the development of a decerebrate rigidity. When the cavernous sinus is occluded by an infective process, the contents of the sinus are involved with a resultant cranial nerve paralysis of the third, fourth, and sixth cranial nerves, loss of pain and temperature sensation in the distribution of the first branch of the trigeminal nerve, and occasionally an occlusion of the internal carotid artery. In cavernous sinus thrombosis there is also proptosis and edema of the eye.

In the treatment of dural sinus thrombosis, therapy is aimed at the underlying cause and at relieving the occlusive. If infection is the cause, the energetic and proper use of chemotherapeutic and antibiotic agents is indicated. The maintenance of proper fluid and electrolyte balance is important. When the sinus is amenable to surgical approach (for example, the lateral or superior sagittal sinuses), surgical evacuation is indicated. When it is not (for example, the vein of Galen) or after surgical therapy, anticoagulation with heparin followed by dicumarol is indicated.

CEREBRAL HEMORRHAGE

Cerebral hemorrhage is a massive bleeding into the substance of the brain and rarely primarily into the ventricular system.

The **etiology** of cerebral hemorrhage is usually based on arteriosclerotic hypertension. The exact mechanism by which the bleeding occurs is open to some question as to whether it is due to erosion of the vessel wall by atheromatous plaques or to previous softening of the brain tissues surrounding the artery and aneurysmal dilatation resulting from the arteriosclerotic plaque formation. This is academic because certainly the hemorrhage is due to the rupture of a vessel of appreciable size with the free flowing of blood into the brain tissue. Cerebral hemorrhage may also occur, even as an early sign, from infected emboli, such as in patients with subacute bacterial endocarditis; it occurs as a terminal event in patients with blood dyscrasias, particularly in those with leukemia, and occurs from vascular anomalies such as hemangiomas within the substance of the brain.

The **clinical signs** of cerebral hemorrhage caused by arteriosclerotic hypertension are as follows. The patients generally show other evidences of cardiovascular renal disease. The onset is abrupt and occurs when the patient is active and is usually without prodromas of headaches or transient neurologic deficits and signs. Cerebral hemorrhage is generally accompanied by early disturbance in consciousness, which becomes progressively deeper; the patient passes into a coma in a matter of minutes or hours. The neurologic signs such as hemiplegia may begin in one part such as the arm and spread as the hemorrhage grows. The same is true of speech disturbances and sensory or other manifestations. There is often nuchal rigidity and a positive Kernig's sign because of blood in the subarachnoid space. As the patient sinks into deeper coma, the evidence of respiratory involvement and brain stem involvement becomes apparent with respiratory irregularities and bilateral pyramidal tract signs.

Important **laboratory studies** include the cerebrospinal fluid examination. The spinal fluid is bloody and is under increased intracranial pressure in 80% of the patients. There is also a leukocytosis on examination of the blood.

The various scanning techniques, isotope and especially CT, give an early assessment of the location and extent of the hemorrhage.

The **treatment** of cerebral hemorrhage is largely supportive. The use of pharmacologic agents to depress the blood pressure levels and the use of hypothermia may hold some possibility of decreasing the blood flow to the critical level, although this is still in an experimental stage.

Occasionally a patient in the younger age group will improve in 24 to 48 hours and will seem to be recovering. Then after a three- to four-day period, he will begin again to sink into deeper unconsciousness, with more severe increase in his neurologic signs. At this time brain stem signs begin to appear. Such patients have an encapsulated hematoma. Surgical evacuation of the clot is indicated if their general physical condition warrants.

SUBARACHNOID HEMORRHAGE

The most common **cause** of hemorrhage into the interstitial spaces of the pia arachnoid is rupture of a congenital aneurysm. Trauma and a rupture into the subarachnoid space of an intracerebral hemorrhage also produce this picture. Congenital intracranial aneurysms occur in the circle of Willis, predominantly in the anterior portion. Their presence may be evidenced without rupture by the appearance of headache and nerve palsies, particularly of the oculomotor and abducens nerves. However, most aneurysms are first evidenced by rupture and the extravasation of blood into the subarachnoid space.

The **clinical signs** of subarachnoid hemorrhage caused by a ruptured aneurysm appear abruptly, often when the patient is in some period of activity. The onset is with severe excruciating headache followed rather quickly by nuchal rigidity and disturbances of consciousness, and depending on the site of the aneurysm, possible cranial nerve palsies. After the blood has been present in the spinal fluid for an hour or so, low-grade fever appears. The diagnosis of subarachnoid hemorrhage is made by lumbar puncture and the finding of bloody spinal fluid usually under increased pressure.

Arteriography is of the utmost importance in determining the presence and location of an aneurysm. Not all aneurysms, however, are evident on arteriography, and indeed, shortly after rupture the aneurysm may be obscured by spasm of the parent vessel in the neighborhood of the aneurysm. Arteriography is mandatory in patients with subarachnoid hemorrhage, to determine, if possible, the location of the aneurysm and the best possible approach in management of the patient. There is still some difference of opinion concerning how soon arteriography should be performed. If a patient is in desperate straits, obviously the study must be done as a means of indicating a possible lifesaving procedure. If not, it is possible to wait until the initial period of three or four days is past. However, this leaves one vulnerable, for the second subarachnoid hemorrhage that so often follows within a week or ten days of the original onset is frequently fatal.

HEMANGIOMAS AND ARTERIOVENOUS ANEURYSMS

There are relatively rare vascular anomalies, such as hemangiomas and large arteriovenous aneurysms. Since the advent of arteriography, however, the hemangiomas are found to be more common than we formerly believed. These are collections of abnormal vessels that have been present since the formation of the blood supply of the brain. The hemangiomas may be situated in any location but are more common over the parietal lobe and on the bank of the sylvian fissure. They often are wedge shaped, with the base of the triangle at the cortex and the apex directly toward the white matter, and may be arteriovenous and have sinusoids. **Clinically,** they may evidence themselves by repeated small vascular accidents all in the same location, becoming progressively worse, or may present a clinical picture of subarachnoid hemorrhage, although the latter is less common. Various kinds of epileptic phenomena may also be the presenting symptoms.

Among the congenital arteriovenous aneurysms are those peculiar rare anomalies involving the great vein of Galen, the straight sinus, and aberrant arteries from the circle of Willis.

VASCULAR DISEASE OF THE SPINAL CORD

In contradistinction to vascular involvement of the brain, impairment of circulation to the spinal cord is rare indeed. **Transverse myelitis** due to arteriosclerosis with the syndrome of acute transection of the cord is rare. **Occlusion of the anterior spinal artery** is the most common vascular disease of the cord, but it, too, is infrequent. In this syndrome the ventral and

lateral columns and the anterior horns of the cord become softened. Clinically the onset is acute, often is associated with excess activity in older patients, and presents with weakness and
pyramidal tract signs in both legs and loss of pain and temperature sensation below the level of the lesion. Anterior horn cell
signs can be demonstrated, with care, at the level of the lesion.
Syphilitic meningomyelitis causing a bilateral spastic paraplegia is rare.

OTHER VASCULAR DISEASES OF THE NERVOUS SYSTEM

Mention has been made previously of the **collagenous diseases** as a rare but definite cause of cerebrovascular disease.
These diseases, with their peculiar involvement of blood vessels, may involve the spinal cord also in extremely rare cases.
More commonly, however, especially in periarteritis nodosa,
the blood vessels of the peripheral nerves may be involved,
with a resultant neuritis. This may be a mononeuritis, a multiple neuritis (that is, involvement of more than one peripheral
nerve, such as the radial nerve on one side and the ulnar on the
other), or a polyneuritis (with essentially distal motor and sensory involvement).

REHABILITATION THERAPY

Rehabilitation consists of teaching the patient to employ the
undamaged portions of the nervous system, but it will not re-
construct the various speech areas or the corticospinal pathway. Fortunately in the organization of the central nervous
system there is some overlap of function. This was demonstrated by Fulton and his colleagues for the parietal lobe,
at first in subhuman primates and later in humans.

Since rehabilitation is a learning process, it is necessary to
begin therapy as soon as possible and before the patient has
acquired undesirable methods of handling the deficit. Therapy
should begin as soon as the patient is conscious and out of
danger. Passive exercises and appropriate placing of the

paralyzed parts are a simple beginning for the bedfast patient.

Rehabilitation therapy requires a team effort, including the appropriate physician, physical therapist, occupational therapist, and when speech is involved, speech therapist. Access to an appropriate prosthetic shop is a distinct advantage.

A most important, if not the most important member of the team, is the patient. And his family is only a little less important! Patient motivation is essential, and this is best acquired early. Family efforts need to be supportive but not smothering!

PREVENTION OF CEREBROVASCULAR ACCIDENTS

The most important aspect of therapy is prevention! Cerebrovascular disease has a high mortality and a devastating morbidity, it is treated by drastic methods, both medical and surgical in the acute phases, and rehabilitative therapy still leaves much to be desired.

Age is an important factor in the development of strokes. This cannot be altered, but middle-aged and older persons should be checked periodically for stroke-inducing factors, the most important of which is hypertension. Diabetes, so often associated with arteriosclerosis, is another factor. Cardiac disorders are associated with emboli, as noted before, and appropriate treatment is indicated. The role of serum lipid elevation is unclear, but elevations of cholesterol in individuals under the age of 50 years may be significant. Obesity, not related to other factors, is apparently unimportant, but cigarette smoking seems to increase the risk of cerebral infarction.

It is therefore especially important for the primary physician to advise his patients, with the hope of preventing these catastrophic illnesses.

REFERENCES

Brock, M., et al., editors: Cerebral blood flow, New York, 1969, Springer-Verlag, New York, Inc.

Fields, W. S.: Pathogenesis and treatment of cerebrovascular diseases, Springfield, Ill., 1961, Charles C Thomas, Publisher.

Fulton, J. F.: Physiology of the nervous system, ed. 3, New York, 1949, Oxford University Press.

Kubik, C. S., and Adams, R. D.: Occlusion of the basilar artery: clinical and pathological study, Brain **69:**73, 1946.

Marshall, J.: The management of cerebrovascular disease, London, 1965, J. & A. Churchill, Ltd.

Masucci, E. F.: Bilateral ophthalmoplegia in basilar-vertebral artery disease, Brain **88:**97, 1965.

Millikan, C. H., Siekert, R. G., and Whisnant, J. P.: Cerebral vascular diseases, Transactions of the Fourth Conference, New York, 1965, Grune & Stratton, Inc.

Report of the Ad Hoc Committee of the N.I.N.D.B.: A classification and outline of cerebrovascular disease, Neurology (Minneap.) **8:**1, 1958.

Sahs, A. L., Hartman, E. C., and Aronson, S. M., editors: Guide lines for stroke care, DHEW pub. no. (HRA) [76–1]4017, Washington, D.C., 1976, Government Printing Office.

Toole, J. F., Moosy, J., and Janeway, J.: Cerebral vascular disease, Seventh Conference, New York, 1971, Grune & Stratton, Inc.

Toole, J. F., Siekert, R. G., and Whisnant, J. P.: Cerebral vascular disease, Sixth Conference, New York, 1968, Grune & Stratton, Inc.

Wright, I. S., and Millikan, C. H.: Cerebral vascular diseases, Third Conference, New York, 1962, Grune & Stratton, Inc.

5 Headache

Before considering headache from the clinical standpoint, it is necessary to note the cranial pain-sensitive structures and the basic mechanisms for the production of headache.

The **cranial pain-sensitive structures** are the coverings of the skull, including the periosteum and skin, the dura at the base of the skull, the dural venous sinuses and their large tributaries, the branches of the fifth, ninth, and tenth cranial nerves and of the first to the third cervical nerves, and the large arteries at the base of the brain. Pain can be elicited from the sensitive structures by traction on the dura, displacement of the venous sinuses, traction on the middle meningeal arteries, traction on the large arteries at the base of the brain, distention and displacement of the large arteries, direct pressure on the fifth, ninth, and tenth cranial nerves or on the first to the third cervical nerves, or inflammation about any of the pain-sensitive structures.

In addition to these mechanisms are certain referred pains from the other cranial structures—the paranasal sinuses, the mastoid air cells, the muscles of the scalp and neck, and the external ocular muscles.

MIGRAINE

Migraine is an ancient clinical entity. The **etiology** of these headaches and the associated symptoms are somewhat paradoxical. The headache itself is due to vasodilatation involving the extracerebral arteries, both intracranial and extracranial, and particularly involving the middle meningeal arteries and the branches of the temporal arteries. Thermography, the photographic demonstration of emission of radiant heat, and cutaneous blood flow studies show that the peripheral blood flow in the area of the headache is increased. The central nervous system features, such as visual disturbances, are characteristic of vasospasms. The arteries involved in vasospasm are the intracerebral arteries. This clinical impression is supported by evidence derived from angiography and cerebral blood flow studies using inhalation of radioactive xenon. The possibility has been raised that the cerebral manifestations are due to a spreading depression of the electrical activity of the cortex. The possible role of humoral factors in the causation of migraine has evoked considerable interest, and at present it appears that at least three biochemical keys are in operation: noradrenaline, serotonin, and bradykinin. At this time there is no convincing evidence that histamine or acetylcholine plays a significant role.

Migraine may present in various forms but the best defined is the classic form. Somewhat less typical is the common migraine, and hemiplegic and ophthalmoplegic forms are uncommon. Cluster headache is a special type of migraine.

CLASSIC MIGRAINE

Certain cardinal **clinical features** should be present before the diagnosis of classic migraine is established. The most important of these are (1) a positive family history, (2) the characteristic unilateral headache, (3) associated visual phenomena, and (4) associated gastrointestinal disturbances. In addition to these, the onset of the headache should be in the second or third decade of life. Seldom does migraine have its onset later than the third decade, and even when the onset is late in the third decade, suspicion of another cause for the periodic headaches is warranted.

The **positive family history** of migraine occurs on the maternal side in a ratio of 3:1. It is not sufficient, however, to have a family history of headaches—familial headaches should also be migraine in type.

The **characteristics** of the migraine **headache** are the unilaterality, the throbbing nature, and occurrence on either side in different attacks. The assumption that migraine is the cause of unilateral headaches which occur always on the same side is open to grave doubt, since these may be due to a vascular anomaly, such as an aneurysm.

Visual disturbances often precede the headache and may vary from visual blurring that is not sharply defined to a distinct homonymous hemianopia. More frequent, however, is scotoma, often flashing and beginning in a whirling fashion. Sometimes a parapet type of scotoma manifests itself in a zigzag fashion much like the rampart of a medieval castle. Minor ocular symptoms include photophobia. During a headache, patients with migraine turn out the light indoors, lower the blinds, and prefer to remain in the dark.

The **gastroenteric disturbances** associated with migraine are nausea and vomiting. Some patients are relieved of their headache after the vomiting. It is the gastrointestinal disturbances of these headaches that have given rise to the layman's term "sick headaches."

Among other **minor associated factors** is tenderness of the scalp. Often during the episode patients cannot comb their hair. Hyperacusis is frequent in attacks. Patients also turn off the radio and are irritated by the normal noise of their children.

The migraine attacks are **episodic** and vary in their frequency and duration from patient to patient. Rarely will a patient have more than one headache a week. Usually the incidence is one every two weeks to one a month. The duration of headaches varies from a few hours to several days. In some patients the attacks are so severe and prolonged that the free intervals are much less than the headache periods.

Most patients who have migraine headaches are rigid and perfectionistic in their **personalities,** are precise in all their activities, and are disturbed by the miscarriage of plans even to a relatively mild degree. Their lives are often disturbed by the headache, and all arrangements in their daily planning are made contingent on "whether they have a headache."

In the **common migraine** the **clinical picture** is not as clear cut. The headaches are unilateral, are not preceded by neurologic signs, often are noted on waking, and may last all day until the patient returns to sleep. Rhinorrhea may occur on the side of the headache. Although the headaches are accompanied or followed by other symptoms, these also are not as clearly defined as in the classic form of migraine. The symptoms may be vague such as chilliness, polyuria, lassitude, and occasionally photophobia and hyperacusis.

Rare forms of migraine are characterized by transient neurologic deficits. In some patients transient paralyses of the extraocular muscles occur (ophthalmoplegic migraine), and some patients have transient hemiplegia accompanied by aphasia when the dominant side is involved (hemiplegic migraine). A rare form, basilar artery migraine, occurs in young women and consists of bilateral visual field defects followed by vertigo, ataxia, dysarthria, paresthesias of the extremities, and even loss of consciousness. The duration of the episode is less than a half hour.

The **medical treatment** of migraine consists of the use of specific preparations at the time of the attack and preventive measures at other times. In the acute attack ergotamine tartrate may be used orally in doses of 5 mg at the onset of the headache and 1 or 2 mg/hr for 3 hours succeeding onset, to a total dosage of 8 to 11 mg for a given headache.

Caffeine has long been a favorite home remedy for migraine, and the combination of caffeine and ergotamine is often valuable. This combination may be employed in tablets containing 1 mg of ergotamine and 100 mg of caffeine (Cafergot). These tablets may be given in doses of two at the onset of the headache and one every half hour, until a total dosage of six tablets has been administered.

If the oral administration of the ergotamine preparations is not feasible because of vomiting, the suppository or inhalation preparations can be employed. When the oral and rectal routes of administration fail to abort the headaches, intramuscular or intravenous administration can be tried. Ergotamine tartrate itself may be administered parenterally in 1 ml ampules, the dose being 0.5 ml intramuscularly or intravenously. If no relief has been obtained in 20 to 30 minutes, this 0.5 ml dose may be repeated. Dihydroergotamine tartrate (DHE) may be employed in 0.5 to 2 mg dosage intramuscularly or intravenously. Ergotamine or DHE may also be employed parenterally as a therapeutic test in a definite attack and before oral administration is prescribed, leading to a firm establishment of the diagnosis. The ergot preparations are effective only when given in the early phases of the migraine attack. The administration of these drugs is ineffectual once the migraine attack becomes well established.

These ergotamine preparations cannot be given with impunity. They are contraindicated in patients with cardiovascular or renal diseases. In pregnancy they should be used judiciously, and then dihydroergotamine tartrate is preferable. The ergotamines cannot be given too frequently and should never be employed as preventives. The use of ergotamine in daily doses to avoid migraine headaches is not justified. A person should never be given ergot preparations more often than once every two weeks for headaches. Patients who have more frequent headaches may choose which headache they wish to abort and use less effective analgesic agents (for example, the salicylates and phenacetin) for the headaches not to be treated with ergot.

Preventive measures include a reconsideration of the patient's attitude toward environment and particularly the patient's role in it. In addition to these psychotherapeutic measures, a serotonin antagonist, methysergide (Sansert), has been successfully employed. Taken in daily doses of 4 to 6 mg, this drug often prevents the attacks. Sansert, a serotonin inhibitor, may inhibit the activity of mast cells. Prolonged usage may lead to peripheral vascular insufficiency or to retroperitoneal fibrosis. This is therefore not a safe drug for prolonged use but may be effective for short-term therapy by producing a change in the pattern of frequency, thus permitting reduction and stoppage of the drug.

Many patients with migraine are also subject to depression. Amitriptyline (Elavil) therefore was first employed to offset the depression and thus alter the headache incidence. It is now apparent that this is the drug of choice for the prevention of migraine headaches and that the salutary effect is not due to the antidepressant action.

In general, the daily administration of ergotamine preparations as a preventive measure is considered dangerous. However, when necessary, relatively small doses of ergot usually in combination with other medications may prove successful. The combination of ergot, phenobarbital, and belladonna (Bellergal) can be administered.

Patients with anxiety and difficulty in handling the stresses of daily living may derive prophylactic aid from the use of barbiturates, phenothiazine derivatives, and the minor tranquilizers.

Migraine may be induced or aggravated by the use of anovulatory contraceptive measures. In the prevention of attacks it is often necessary for the patient to stop taking these preparations.

CLUSTER HEADACHES

Cluster headaches are more common in men than in women and consist of a series of headaches occurring in rapid succession over a period of days or weeks, followed by a free period of weeks, months, or even years. The headache itself is similar to that of migraine, but prodromes are uncommon, and nasal stuffiness, tearing, and flushing of the face, especially on the involved side are often associated. Whether this is a form of migraine is not clear. Formerly these headaches were attributed to histamine sensitization, but this is no longer considered valid.

TEMPORAL ARTERITIS

Temporal arteritis is not a frequent cause of headache, but it is most important that it be diagnosed and treated promptly. Pathologically there is inflammation with giant cell formation in the walls of the temporal artery, but intracranial arteries are also involved. The disease occurs in older patients of either sex. The headache is severe and localized in the region of the temporal artery, which is often palpably thickened, may be nodular, and is tender. General symptoms such as anorexia and fever often occur. The diagnosis is made by the clinical picture and can usually be confirmed by the presence of leukocytosis, increased sedimentation rate, or biopsy of the artery. When the diagnosis is made, ACTH or steroid therapy should be instituted promptly, not only for the relief of pain but especially to prevent involvement of the ophthalmic artery, leading to blindness, or of the intracranial arteries with a resultant cerebrovascular accident.

HYPERTENSIVE HEADACHES

Headache is not a prominent part of the picture in mild hypertension, at least not until the diagnosis of hypertension is made. The headache of mild hypertension is not characteristic and may be of either the migraine or tension type. In severe hypertension frequent and intense headaches may occur, are usually occipital, and are present on waking. When these headaches are pulsatile, and especially if associated with tachycardia, pallor, nausea, and vomiting, the possibility of a pheochromocytoma should be considered.

Since the severity of hypertensive headaches is related to the severity of the hypertension, the obvious therapy is to treat the hypertension, either by removing the cause when this is feasible, for example, pheochromocytoma, or by symptomatic therapy.

HEADACHES SECONDARY TO NASAL AND PARANASAL DISEASE

The mucous membrane of the turbinates, ostia, and ducts of the sinuses is six times more sensitive than that of the sinuses themselves. The sinusal mucosa is only as sensitive as the surfaces of the tongue.

The location of the headache gives some indication of which sinus is involved. Headache due to inflammation in the superior group of sinuses is felt on the anterior portion of the head and in and between the eyes, whereas those headaches arising from the middle and inferior sinuses are felt over the zygomas, temples, teeth, and jaws. The headaches caused by sinusitis are increased by bending forward and are constant, dull, and moderately severe in comparison with those of migraine or brain tumor. Whenever a young patient complains of a sharp lancinating pain over the side of the face that resembles tic douloureux, the nasal sinuses and teeth should be especially screened for the etiologic agent of the headache.

OCULAR HEADACHES

Increase in intraocular tension, such as that occurring in patients with glaucoma, gives rise to a sharp headache that is radiated over the ophthalmic branch of the fifth cranial nerve. Muscular imbalance, astigmatism, and hyperopia produce tenseness, heaviness, and a headache that occurs periorbitally and radiates to the occiput. The occipital headache often results from contraction of the scalp and neck muscles. Myopia itself seldom causes severe headaches.

The **characteristics** of ocular headache are definite. They are not present on awakening, occur with use of the eyes, and are relieved by rest. These traits, coupled with the location of the headache, indicate their ocular origin. A rare cause of this ocular type of headache is a reading difficulty, either an acquired alexia, as in an aphasic patient, or more commonly a congenital alexia. The constant strain of attempted reading may produce an ocular type of headache that is not improved by the use of glasses.

TENSION HEADACHES

Tension headaches are derived from the sustained contraction of muscles of the scalp and neck. They may occur as an entity by themselves and then are usually associated with poorly maintained posture, either as a part of an occupation or more commonly as a complication of psychic tension. Constant psychic tension can also produce a generalized headache, with or without a vascular component. Moreover, this type of headache may complicate other types of headache. Many patients with migraine, after relieving their throbbing headache by taking ergotamine or similar preparations, are left with a residual aching, dull headache mostly over the occiput. Therefore the tension headache component is still present.

Tension headache can be relieved by improving posture, by the administration of muscle relaxant drugs and ataractic agents, and by the application of heat to the affected muscles. Biofeedback mechanisms can be employed successfully in the treatment of tension headaches. The patient is presented with a visual or auditory display of the electromyogram of the involved muscles. The patient can be taught to control the contractions and relax the muscles. Adjustment to the pertinent life situation is of great importance in tension headache patients.

POSTTRAUMATIC HEADACHE

Posttraumatic headache is a difficult problem occurring after cerebral concussion. It is dull, often poorly described, and usually generalized. Some feelings of dizziness, giddiness, and emotional instability generally accompany the posttraumatic headache. In its full-blown state, memory difficulty also occurs. This is actually a description of the posttraumatic syndrome, and the headache is only a component of it. The syndrome occurs after concussion rather than after focal brain damage. It tends to disappear within six months in 75% of the patients and within two years in about 95% of the patients.

There is often a considerable functional component. Difficulty in diagnosis is proportional to the degree to which functional elements contribute to the clinical syndrome.

LUMBAR PUNCTURE HEADACHE

One of the simplest headaches to understand is that due to lumbar puncture (known also as the spinal drainage headache, postspinal fluid drainage headache, or the postlumbar puncture headache). The lumbar puncture headache is produced by spinal fluid leakage through the puncture holes in the dura and arachnoid. The fluid is absorbed from the muscles of the back. In an ordinary lumbar puncture a patient has an initial spinal fluid pressure of 150 mm H_2O, and after 8 to 10 ml of spinal fluid are removed, the patient is left with a final pressure of 90 mm H_2O. If the puncture holes through the arachnoid and the dura are superimposed on removal of the needle, it is possible for the spinal fluid to leak through these superimposed apertures. The spinal fluid is absorbed in clysis fashion from the muscles of the back. Therefore the spinal fluid pressure is not 90 mm H_2O but is considerably lower than that because of the drainage of the fluid, and this headache is produced by torsion on the venous sinuses.

The lumbar puncture headache appears on the first to third day after the lumbar puncture and lasts for a period of time varying from one to seven days. Usually it disappears between the second and the fourth days, and only rarely does it last longer than a week.

The headache is **characteristic.** It is a severe, pulling, aching kind of headache located over the vertex, often radiating down both sides of the neck into the shoulder. The headache is aggravated by coughing, sneezing, or jugular compression. It appears within a few minutes after the erect position is assumed and disappears when the patient lies flat.

The **treatment** of the lumbar puncture headache consists in maintaining the patient in a recumbent position without a pillow for 24 to 36 hours after the onset of the headache, forcing fluids, and liberally using caffeine, either in a palatable beverages such as coffee or, if necessary, in tablet form. In an acute situation when it is necessary for a patient to to journey a relatively short distance by car, it is possible to relieve the post-lumbar puncture headache by intravenous injection of caffeine sodium benzoate ($3^3/_4$ grams) to allow the patient to return home in comfort before resuming the recumbent position.

BRAIN TUMOR HEADACHE

The headaches of brain tumor were long considered to be the result of an actual increase of intracranial pressure—now known to be a fallacious concept, since the occurrence of headache and increased intracranial pressure cannot be well correlated. Patients with headache, brain tumors, and increased intracranial pressure may have their intracranial hypertension decreased without relief of the headache. Some patients with brain tumors have headaches prior to a demonstrable increase in intracranial pressure. The mechanism of headache in brain tumor is distortion of pain-sensitive structures at least in the early phases, and later the increase in intracranial pressure may cause distortion of pain-sensitive structures at a distance from the actual site of the lesion. Thus traction on pain-sensitive structures directly caused by the tumor produces early headache of fairly accurate localizing value. This is almost always on the same side of the head as the tumor, and in approximately two thirds of the patients this early headache overlies a brain tumor.

The headaches of brain tumor themselves are not characteristic. They vary from relatively mild to excruciatingly sharp headaches, which make the patient lie with his head over the side of the bed and scream with pain. The severity and character of the headache are in themselves not criteria for the determination of the presence of brain tumor. There is some exception, however, in that the headache of posterior fossa tumor, particularly the early headache, usually is occipital and is associated with tenderness of the calvarium.

REFERENCES

Bickerstaff, E. R.: Basilar artery migraine, Lancet **1:**15, 1961.

Friedman, A. P., and Elkind, A. H.: Appraisal of methysergide in the treatment of vascular headaches of the migraine type, J.A.M.A. **184:**125, 1963.

Friedman, A. P., and Frazier, S. H.: The headache book, New York, 1973, Dodd, Mead & Co., Inc.

Friedman, A. P., and Losin, S.: Evaluation of UML-491 in the treatment of vascular headaches, Arch. Neurol. **4:**241, 1961.

Friedman, A. P., and Merritt, H. H.: Headache—diagnosis and treatment, Philadelphia, 1959, F. A. Davis Co.

Graham, J. R., Suby, H. L., Le Compte, P. R., and Sadowsky, N. L.: Fibrotic disorders associated with methysergide therapy, N. Engl. J. Med. **274:** 359, 1966.

Neurology, special issue, March, 1963, p. 44.

Research and clinical studies in headache: an international review, vol. I, Basel, 1967, S. Karger, A.G.

Sicuteri, F.: Mast cells and their active substances: their role in the pathogenesis of migraine, Headache **3:**86, 1963.

Wolff, H. G.: Headaches and other head pain, ed. 2, New York, 1963, Oxford University Press.

6 Epilepsy

The epilepsies, in view of incidence and chronicity, constitute one of the most important areas in the entire field of neurology. The term "epilepsy" merely means that the patient has seizures but does not connote the cause of the seizures.

The **incidence** of epilepsy is close to 1% of the population, or approximately 2 million epileptics, in the United States. Seizures occur in members of all races and in all geographic areas, and the incidence is approximately the same in each sex.

Etiology

The etiology of epilepsy is complex. Almost every known disease of the nervous system and, indeed, many systemic diseases have been described as producing seizures. In addition to this is the fact that patients may have seizures as a disease sui generis, that is, on a **genetic, inherited** basis. With the advances in research, the proportion of patients with so-called idiopathic (genetic, essential, or centrencephalic) epilepsy has become increasingly less, and that of patients with symptomatic epilepsy has become greater.

Among diseases causing seizures, those producing atrophic lesions of the cerebral hemispheres are the most common. They may originate in the antenatal or perinatal period and therefore may result from malformations, failure of development of the blood supply to the particular part of the brain, accidents of birth, or problems of hypoxia in the perinatal and early antenatal period. Atrophic lesions also may result from **trauma** at birth, due to molding of the head and marked herniation of the brain, or from trauma in later life produced by direct head injuries. Therefore seizures are a prominent part of the clinical picture in cerebral palsy. Atrophic lesions may result from vascular accidents that occur during febrile episodes in childhood **(febrile thromboses).** However, seizures are uncommon as a sequela of vascular accidents later in life. Atrophic lesions may occur in the course of a **degenerative disease** in childhood (such as Schilder's disease) or in later life (such as Alzheimer's or Pick's disease).

In patients with **brain tumors,** seizures are a prominent and indeed often the only clinical manifestation. Ths appearance of seizures after the age of 20 years immmediately raises this diagnostic possibility. The type of seizures in patients with brain tumors depends on the location of the neoplasm.

Metabolic errors, both inborn and acquired, are more common causes of seizures in infancy and childhood. Phenylketonuria, Tay-Sachs disease, and Niemann-Pick disease are the most important of the inborn errors, whereas hypo-glycemia, hypocalcemia, and vitamin B_6 deficiency are usually nonfamilial. **Inflammatory diseases** are a relatively uncommon cause of seizures in Europe and North America. However, in some parts of the world parasitic infections such as schistosomiasis and echinococcus are prominent etiologic agents. Brain abscess is not a common disease, and seizures are not a significant part of the clinical picture, especially after the acute phase.

Although the incidence and mortality of bacterial meningitis has decreased survival, particularly with the development of significant cerebromeningeal scarring, this disease may cause seizures.

Seizures are a prominent part in the clinical picture of certain encephalitides. Convulsions can occur after immunizations, especially those for smallpox and tetanus. They occur during the febrile response to the vaccination and usually when the patients are in the first year of life and they may lead to future seizures of various types. This morbidity has led to the discontinuance of smallpox vaccination in infancy.

Whereas central nervous system syphilis is at the present time uncommon, the rising incidence of primary syphilis makes it likely that, unfortunately, the later and therefore central nervous system manifestations will again become evident. Seizures are a prominent part of the clinical picture of central nervous system syphilis, especially generalized paresis. Seizures are also a symptom of disturbances of the nutrition of the cerebral cortex and are common in the clinical picture of proline deficiency.

Seizures occur in chronic alcoholism, especially in the patients with poor nutrition and hygiene, and most frequently occur as a withdrawal symptom. Seizures may also occur with the abrupt withdrawal of sedatives, especially the barbiturates. Also, the administration of certain medications such as the tricyclic antidepressants and phenothiazines in somewhat rare instances may evoke seizures. Disease causing a significant decrease in cerebral blood flow, particularly when the decrease is acute, may also produce seizures. Another cause of seizures is disturbance of cardiac rhythm, as in patients with heart block or carotid sinus hypersensitivity.

Clinical aspects

The clinical types of epileptic seizures are varied. The most pronounced seizure is the **generalized convulsion (grand mal seizure,** or **major motor convulsion).** It may or may not be preceded by an aura. The seizure itself begins with a cry preceding loss of consciousness and tonic stiffening of the body followed by clonic movements of all four extremities, the face, jaw, and head. After the seizure is a prolonged period of unconsciousness. During the attack the patient may bite his tongue, experience urinary incontinence, and sustain injuries in a fall. The entire seizure lasts from 3 to 5 minutes and is followed by a period of coma or deep stupor. On arousing from the coma, the patient is usually achy, has a headache, and may vomit.

A **generalized major motor seizure** may actually have a strong **focal component,** which implies that one area of the

brain is the source for the seizure discharge. This focal component may occur in the aura, in the mode of onset, or in the postictal state of the patient. If the patient's aura is truly
nonspecific, that is, a vague feeling of an impending seizure,
there is no particular indication of specificity. If, however, the
patient's aura includes focal neurophysiologic phenomena
such as scintillating scotoma in one visual field, auditory hallucination (buzzing, words, or music), paresthesias in one arm
or leg, or a vivid recall of a previously experienced condition,
each of these indicates a particular area of the cortex as the
focus for the onset of the seizure. If the onset of the seizures is
always characterized by head and eye deviation to one side or
rotation of the trunk and head to the same side, this indicates a
lesion in the opposite hemisphere, usually in the frontal or temporal lobe. After a single seizure the presence of unilateral
weakness, sensory changes, speech defect, or visual field defect in the postictal state suggests that the area of cortex from
which the seizure had its origin is in a period of decreased activity (Todd's paralysis). This, too, is indicative of focal onset
for the seizures.

Petit mal attacks are the minor seizures occurring in children, usually at a frequency of more than one a day and often
as many as several hundred a day, with each attack lasting less
than 1 minute. These seizures are characterized by a short star-
ing episode (petit mal absence), which may be associated with
myoclonic jerks (myoclonic petit mal attacks). In some patients the petit mal seizures are even shorter in duration and
may consist of only a quick, sudden dropping of objects or falling to the floor (akinetic petit mal seizures). These akinetic attacks may last only a fraction of a second. In true petit mal seizures the electroencephalographic pattern is characteristically
a three per second wave and spike dysrhythmia that is
bilaterally synchronous and occurs over the entire brain. These
dysrhythmias, however, are often somewhat atypical—the
rate is somewhat faster than three per second; the spikes may
be multiple and not bilaterally symmetrical. The dysrhythmia

may then be suspected to originate from one or more foci, often cortical, firing into the reticular formation and by way of this synchronizing network being relayed back to both hemispheres.

Partial complex seizures (automatism, psychomotor seizures, or epileptic fugue states) are attacks characterized by involuntary purposeful but irrelevant activity for which the patient has an amnesia. In these attacks patients can walk, drive a car, or carry out with their hands or feet complex actions that are purposeful but out of contact with the reality of the situation. An example of this is a school teacher who taught civics in high school. During the playing of the national anthem in the school convocation, he failed to rise, moved restlessly in his chair, and cursed audibly above the music. These attacks are often preceded or accompanied by movements of the lips and tongue or gurgling noises. Their duration may be from 3 to 5 minutes. Electroencephalographic tracings are characterized by a temporal lobe spike dysrhythmia that may be observed in the interseizure tracing.

Jacksonian motor seizures are focal motor attacks caused by lesions of the motor area of the cerebral cortex. They are characterized by clonic movements and begin in one part and have a highly characteristic march. The most common sites of origin are at the angle of the mouth, in the thumb, and in the great toe. These sites are represented most extensively in the face, hand, and foot areas of the motor cortex. The attacks begin in one part and spread. They may progress over only part of the extremity or face, or they may proceed to involve the entire side. In Jacksonian seizures no disturbance of consciousness occurs. Occasionally, however, a Jacksonian motor seizure may progress to a generalized seizure with involement of the opposite side of the body. When this occurs, loss of consciousness ensues.

Jacksonian seizures may be **sensory** rather than motor. The patient with these seizures complains of a dysesthesia beginning again in the same parts—angle of the mouth, thumb, or great toe—and spreading sometimes to involve adjacent parts and gradually to include the entire side. Fortunately, for the purpose of clarification of the patient's status, usually some clonic movements are associated with the sensory seizure, since there is some motor representation in the sensory cortex. The clonic movements make it obvious that the sensory disturbances are seizure manifestations of cortical origin rather than of some other source.

Hallucinatory seizures may occur in any of the special sensory fields. **Uncinate,** or olfactory, seizures are characterized by unusual tastes or odors. These episodes last only a few minutes and are unrelated to the environment. Although the experience is generally described by the patient as one involving taste, it is actually among the modalities of smell, that is, odors rather than the basic taste elements (bitter, sweet, salt, and sour). Usually the olfactory hallucination is an unpleasant one; rarely is it something pleasant such as the fragrance of flowers. The hallucination is indicative of a lesion of the uncus. **Visual hallucinatory seizures** may be flashes of light or well-formed images. **Auditory hallucinatory seizures** may be simply vague noises or more highly elaborated ones, such as the sound of voices or music. The patient who is musically educated may be able to draw the score of the auditory musical hallucination. Occasionally the auditory aura may be hyperacusis or hypoacusis. The hallucinatory seizures may serve as the aura for a generalized one or may constitute the entire seizure.

The **reflex epilepsies** include the sensory-precipitated seizures which are evoked by special or somatic sensory stimulation. The most common are those evoked by intermittent light (photosensitive seizures). Stroboscopic stimulation in the laboratory or intermittent light from the shadows in the environment produce seizures, usually petit mal in type and with an electroencephalographic discharge usually of the three per second wave and spike type. Viewing geometric patterns also will evoke seizures in some patients. Startle epilepsy is evoked by a sudden, unexpected, loud noise. Sensory-evoked seizures produced by tapping a part of the body are the most infrequent of all such seizures. Other reflex epilepsies include reading epilepsy, epilepsy evoked by decision making, and musicogenic epilepsy. In reading epilepsy, jaw jerks occur while the patient is reading, and if the reading is continued, the myoclonic jerks become accentuated and may culminate in a convulsion. Musicogenic epilepsy is very rare. In this type the seizures are evoked by the playing of music of a certain composer, a certain melody or class of melodies, or a specific musical note or combination of notes. Many sensory-evoked, or reflex, epilepsies are amenable to a behavioral, or conditioning, type of therapy. Whereas the sensory-evoked seizures at the present time play a small part numerically in the total picture of epilepsy (one out of sixty-five cases, according to Symonds), their importance from the diagnostic and therapeutic standpoint is obvious.

Diagnosis

The diagnosis of epilepsy depends on the establishment of the presence of seizures, as noted previously. The diagnosis of the cause of the epilepsy is more complex. Seizures of the petit mal type, associated with typical three per second wave and spike dysrhythmia, are the essential, idiopathic, or centrencephalic type of epilepsy. Focal seizures are definitely symptomatic, and the cause of the focal lesion must be established with reasonable certainty. Careful recording of family history of the incidence of epilepsy; personal history (the circumstances surrounding birth and development, presence of severe injuries or illnesses, febrile convulsions, mental development, and any indication of change in the development); and an account of the seizures, combined with the complete neurologic evaluation of the patient, makes it possible usually to arrive at a reasonable diagnosis of the cause of the seizures. The diagnosis can be substantiated by laboratory studies.

The most important **laboratory study** in the evaluation of a patient with epilepsy is the electroencephalogram. The presence of focal abnormalities, when substantiated by repeated testing, indicates a distinct area of the brain from which the seizure manifestations arise. The presence of a generalized dysrhythmia without any focal onset, especially when this is the typical three per second wave and spike dysrhythmia, suggests idiopathic epilepsy. Likewise the consistent demonstration of a focal electroencephalographic (EEG) paroxysmal discharge of spiking nature indicates a focal orign of the seizure and a symptomatic basis for the epilepsy. Since the seizures occur episodically and randomly, EEG recording during a seizure is uncommon. The presence of a normal EEG does not rule out the diagnosis of epilepsy. The yield of positive EEGs can be increased in various ways, repeated recording is one of the simplest. Hyperventilation, or overbreathing, during recording is most effective in eliciting dysrhythmias in patients with petit mal epilepsy. Hyperventilation, however, is also efficacious in patients with focal dysrhythmias, especially in partial complex or psychomotor seizures. The hyperventilation often needs to be vigorous and longer than the customary 3-minute period. Recording during sleep is especially useful in eliciting focal temporal lobe dysrhythmias. Additional electrodes, especially nasopharyngeal electrodes, also aid in demonstrating focal dysrhythmias. Routine radiologic study of the skull only occasionally may be helpful but is mandatory in all patients with seizures. Abnormal deposits of calcium may signal the presence of certain brain tumors. Smallness of one side of the skull with thickening of the calvarium on that side and elevation of the base of the skull on the same side are indications of an atrophic lesion that occurred perinatally or early in life in the involved hemisphere. This substantiates the clinical impression of an atrophic lesion. Radioisotopic brain scanning is a useful tool in determining the presence of brain tumor or vascular anomaly as the cause of epilepsy.

The CT, or CAT, scan (p. 37) is especially valuable, since this procedure can demonstrate the presence of neoplasma and moderately sized or larger atrophic lesions, without great discomfort, pain, or risk. Contrast studies may be necessary to establish a more complete evaluation. Injection of air by either lumbar or ventricular route is efficacious in ruling out brain tumors or demonstrating the presence of an atrophic lesion. Arteriography is helpful in determining whether a vascular anomaly such as hemangioma is the cause of the atrophic lesion and in determining the presence of a brain tumor.

Treatment

The treatment of the patient with seizures may be either surgical or medical. Surgical therapy may be mandatory, for example, for a patient with a subdural hematoma or a brain tumor. Indeed, one is then treating primarily an underlying disease and not the seizures. In patients with generalized dysrhythmia and truly generalized seizures such as petit mal, no surgical therapy is available. In patients with focal seizures caused by an atrophic lesion, there is a possibility of surgical therapy, but adequate medical therapy should be employed first, and this usually suffices.

The medical therapy of epilepsy depends on medications of several classes. Bromides, the first effective medication, are rarely employed and then only in patients with severe allergies to other medications. The other classes of antiepileptic medications are barbiturates, hydantoinates, succinimides, primidone, benzodiazepines, oxazolidines, carbamazepine, and acetazolamide. Acetylurea is seldom used now. Sulthiame (Ospolot) is not available in the United States.

Table 1 summarizes in general the indications and relative toxicity of the various classes of antiepileptic medications. The barbituarates, especially phenobarbital, and sodium valproate have broad efficacy in the various seizure types.

Sodium valproate (Depakene) is the newest addition to the antiepilepsy medications. Whereas it is most effective in treating petit mal seizures and least effective in treating focal motor attacks, it appears to be one of the, if not the, most effective anticonvulsant. It is just coming into general use in the United States.

In generalized major motor seizures the hydantoinates,

Table 1

Type of seizure

Class of medication	Generalized		Partial complex	Other focal	Toxicity
	Major motor	Petit mal			
Barbiturates	+++	+	++	++	0
Sodium valproate	+++	+++	++	+	+−
Hydantoinates	++++	−	+++	+++	+−++
Primidone	++++	+−	++++	+++	+
Carbamazepine	+++	0	++++	+++	++
Succinimides	0	++++	+	0	+
Benzodiazepines	+	+++	++	0	+
Oxazolidines	−	++++	0	0	+++
Acetazolimide	+	++	0	0	0
Acetylurea	0	0	++++	0	++++

+ Indicates efficacy in treatment or degree of toxicity.

0 Indicates no efficacy in treatment or no toxicity.

− Indicates contraindication.

primidone (Mysoline) and carbamazepine, are especially useful. Carbamazepine and primidone take precedence if the major seizures are of focal onset. In generalized seizures of the petit mal type, the succinimides are the first choice, followed by the benzodiazepines and then oxazolidines. Acetazolimide plays a limited role in the treatment of these seizures. In the treatment of partial complex (psychomotor) seizures, carbamazepine and primidone are the preferred medications.

Table 2 presents data regarding the various medications within each class. When more than one preparation is available in a given class, the medication of first preference is marked by an asterisk. In the benzodiazepine group, diazepam (Valium) requires special mention. Diazepam is an effective anticonvulsant but has a very short half-life. It is therefore of limited use for oral administration but, as noted later, is the medication of choice for the parenteral treatment of status epilepticus.

The choice of medications depends on an accurate diagnosis

of seizure type—the selection of a medication which is effective in the treatment of that type of seizure but with consideration of the toxicity of the given medication. This is well exemplified by acetylurea, the last medication in Table 1, which is a highly effective anticonvulsant in treating partial complex seizures but is a very dangerous compound and therefore rarely employed.

Blood level determinations of the various antiepileptic drugs are of considerable value in the long-term management of patients. Table 3 presents the serum levels for the most frequently employed medications. Noncompliance on the part of the patient results in subtherapeutic levels. However, this may also results from failures of absorption of the medication. This can be determined by having the patient observed when medications are administered; if they have been swallowed and seizures still occur and the serum levels are low, malabsorption may be assumed. This can be corrected by either increasing dosages or employing a more soluble form, for example, tablets rather than capsules.

Serum levels also are of value in determining either actual or impending toxicity and may be especially helpful in determining which is the offending one of several medications that the patient is taking. Serum levels, however, should be considered as guides not rules of treatment, and dosages should not be decreased because of slightly high levels when the patient shows no toxic signs and, conversely, need not be increased in the seizure-free patient with a level somewhat below the lower limits of the therapeutic range.

There are **minor complications** in the use of the anticonvulsant drugs, including rash and drowsiness, which can occur with any of the anticonvulsant drugs. The rash is usually seen only early in the course of therapy and remits promptly. With long continuation and high dosage, an acneform rash can appear, especially when the barbiturate series is employed. Drowsiness if more common with the barbiturate series and primidone than with other medication. Cerebellar signs such as

Table 2
Epileptic medication: dosages and complications

Drug group	Trade name	Generic name	Size of preparation
Barbiturates	*Phenobarbital	Phenobarbital	Varies 32, 0.1, and 0.2 mg
	Mebaral	Mephobarbital	
	Gemonil	Metharbital	100 mg
Sodium valproate	Depakene	Sodium valproate	250 mg
Hydantoinates	*Dilantin	Phenytoin	100 mg
			50 mg
	Mesantoin	Mephenytoin	100 mg
	Peganone	Ethotoin	250 and 500 mg
Primidones	Mysoline	Primidone	0.25 and 50 mg
Carbamazepine	Tegretol	Carbamazepine	200 mg
Succinimides	Milontin	Phensuximide	500 mg
	Celontin	Methsuximide	300 mg
	*Zarontin	Ethosuximide	250 mg

*Indicates first choice in the class of medications.

Appearance of preparation	Daily adult dosage in grams		Complications	
	Effective	Maximum	Minor	Major
Varies	0.1	0.4	Drowsiness	None
All three white marked with "W" on obverse; 0.032, pink band; 0.2, three dots and scored; 0.1, one dot	0.3	1.25	Drowsiness	None
White, scored tablet	0.1	0.3	Rash, drowsiness	None
Capsules	15 mg/ kg	30 mg/ kg	Nausea, hair loss, diarrhea	Rare hepatic disease
White capsule with pink or red band (some plain, white capsules only	0.3	0.6	Rash, hypertrichosis, hypertrophic gums, ataxia, diplopia, nystagmus	Rare lymphocyte reaction
Triangular tablet				
Pink, scored tablet	0.4	1.0	Similar to Dilantin	Aplastic anemia, agranulocytosis
Grooved, white tablet	2.0	4.0	Similar to Dilantin	Rare blood dyscrasia
Large, white, scored tablet	0.25	2.0	Drowsiness, vomiting	Drowsiness
Small tablet				
White tablets	200 mg	1,200 mg	Dizziness	Anemia
White capsule, orange band	0.5	3.5	None	None
Yellow capsule, orange band	0.3	1.2	Drowsiness, blurred vision	Rash, periorbital edema
Clear orange capsule	0.25	1.5	Anorexia, headache, insomnia	Aplastic anemia, agranulocytosis, leukopenia

Continued.

Table 2
Epileptic medication: dosages and complications—cont'd

Drug group	Trade name	Generic name	Size of preparation
Benzodiazepines	Valium	Diazepam	(see text, p. 84)
	Tranxene	Clorazepate	3.75 mg
			7.5 mg
			15.0 mg
	Clonopin	Clonazepam	0.5 mg
			1 mg
			2 mg
Oxazolidines-diones	*Tridione	Trimethadione	300 mg
			150 mg
	Paradione	Paramethadione	300 mg
Sulfonamide derivative	Diamox	Acetazolamide	125 mg
			250 mg
Acetylureas	Phenacemide	Phenurone	500 mg

intention tremor, slurred speech, and ataxis occur particularly in patients taking the hydantoinates in higher dosages. Hypertrichosis and hypertrophy of the gums can occur with hydantoinates and primidone. Nausea, vomiting, and diarrhea may be induced by sodium valproate. The administration of the medications with meals and avoidance of carbonated beverages can prevent these complications.

A mild visual complication is hemeralopia, an unusual brightness of vision. This occurs only when the oxazolidines

| Appearance of preparation | Daily adult dosage in grams | | Complications | |
	Effective	Maximum	Minor	Major
Capsules	15 mg	60 mg	Drowsiness	Rare
Tablets	Varies with age		Drowsiness	Rare
White capsule, coconut odor Troche	0.3	2.7	Rash, hemeralopia	Aplastic anemia, agranulocytosis, renal disease
Red perle	0.3	2.7	Rash, hemeralopia	Same as Tridione
White tablets	375–1,200 mg		Anorexia	Acidosis
Large, white, scored tablet	1.5	3.5	Headache, insomnia, anorexia	Psychotic depression, hepatitis, aplastic anemia

are employed and disappears on discontinuance of medication.

More **serious complications** can occur with the use of the anticonvulsant drugs, including relatively rare but extremely important complications of severe lymphoid reactions resembling granulomas and collagenous diseaselike states. The hydantoinates are the most common offenders in this regard. Rarely a fatal dermatologic disease, bullous erythematosis, can occur with the use of the hydantoinate preparations. More commonly, however, blood dyscrasias occur with the oxazolidines,

Table 3
Serum levels of frequently used antiepileptic medications

Medication		Therapeutic ($\mu g/nk$)	Toxic ($\mu g/ml$)
Generic drug	*Trade name*		
Phenytoin	Dilantin	10–20	30
Phenobarbital		20–40	50
Primidone	Mysoline	5–12	12
Trimethadione	Tridione	700*	
Ethosuximide	Zarontin	40–100	125
Carbamazepine	Tegretol	5–12	Not established yet
Valproic acid	Depakene	50–100	Not established yet

*Level of dimethadione.

Mesantoin, carbamazepine, and Phenurone. It is possible that sodium valproate may produce hepatic disease. When temporal lobe seizures are suppressed by medication, severe personality disorders may occur, particularly when suppression of the seizures has been achieved by the use of Phenurone.

There is some statistical evidence that when anticonvulsant medications are administered to pregnant women, a higher than usual incidence of teratogenic defects may result, especially cleft palate and cleft lip. However, the consensus is that the risk to the mother and baby of withdrawal of medication is too great. In general, the hazards of not treating the potential mother are much greater than the possibility of a teratogenic defect.

Status epilepticus

Status epilepticus is a recurrence of seizures in short order without periods of consciousness between seizures. This term usually connotes recurrent grand mal seizures, although status epilepticus may occur in petit mal epilepsy. Probably the epileptic psychosis is actually psychomotor status. Status epilepticus (major seizures occurring in this rapid order) is a major medical emergency, since permanent brain damage or death may occur. Therefore the treatment of this condition must be immediate. The drug of choice is diazepam (Valium), which is administered intravenously at the rate of 5 mg/min, and the dosage required usually ranges between 2 and 20 mg. It is sometimes necessary to repeat the administration at 10- to 20-minute intervals. Since lingual obstruction is possible, an artificial airway should be available. Diazepam is also effective in petit mal status.

Proper management

The **proper management** of the epileptic patient is aimed at controlling the seizures with medication. When this has been maintained for a sufficiently long period (usually several times the previous length of the longest seizure-free interval), a gradual reduction of medication may be initiated. This reduction is accomplished over a period of years, except in patients with petit mal epilepsy, when the seizures occur so frequently that the time course can be considered abbreviated.

Comparison of the EEG is useful in determining the end point and also the rapidity of decreases in medication. Normal EEGs after a long seizure-free period in a patient with previously abnormal records are reassuring. The ultimate goal of treatment is to reduce medication and leave the patient seizure free. However, when the use of medication is unavailing and the patient's seizures are not controlled and when a definite focus has been established by clinical, EEG, and radiologic evidence, surgical excision of the focus may be helpful. Many of the surgically removable foci are in the temporal lobe. It is important to determine before temporal lobectomy not only which hemisphere is dominant in regard to language functions but also in which temporal lobe memory patterns are banked. This is accomplished by the study of the patient in regard to amobarbital language functions and memory during and after the intracarotid injection sodium (Amytal sodium). The EEG is carefully monitored during the test to be certain the drug was administered to only one hemisphere.

Socioeconomic factors are important in the management of the epileptic patient. The presence of epilepsy alone is not a contraindication for marriage. The presence of seizures in one spouse probably raises the likelihood of seizures in the off-spring, but the genetic transmission is far from dominant. In counseling patients regarding offspring, the cause of epilepsy and type of seizures in the patient, as well as the family history and EEGs of both patient and spouse provide valuable information. Many states have adopted automobile drivers' licensing laws permitting the licensing of epileptics after two seizure-free years, even when this freedom has been acquired by the use of anticonvulsant medication. The performances of these drivers are usually far above the average performance of other drivers, and they have fewer accidents. Employment of the epileptic patient has been made considerably easier in states where second-injury clauses have been appended to the workmen's compensation acts. Most colleges will now accept epileptic students whose seizures are reasonably well controlled, and most occupations are open to epileptics.

A psychological factor of great import is his family's fear that the patient will become mentally retarded. This is partly based on the erroneous historic linking of the epileptic and the insane—a false bond that has been severed. Their concern is also based on knowledge of persons in whom severe brain damage resulted in both seizures and mental retardation as well as other neurologic deficits. Often the only diagnosis they have heard in such cases is that of "epilepsy." It is important to realize that the world would be a much duller place to live in if there had been no epileptics—no Dostoevski, no Julius Caesar, no van Gogh, no de Maupassant, no Haydn, to mention only a few.

REFERENCES

Ajmone-Marson, C., and Ralston, B. L.: The epileptic seizure, Springfield, Ill., 1957, Charles C Thomas, Publisher.

Baldwin, M., and Bailey, P., editors: Temporal lobe epilepsy, Springfield, Ill., 1958, Charles C Thomas, Publisher.

Barrow, R. L., and Fabing, H. D.: Epilepsy and the law, New York, 1956, Paul B. Hoeber, Inc., Medical Book Department of Harper & Row, Publishers, Inc.

Epilepsia **18:** June, 1977. (Series of papers on sodium valproate.)

Forster, F. M.: Treatment of epilepsy. In Forster, F. M., editor: Modern therapy in neurology, St. Louis, 1957, The C. V. Mosby Co.

Forster, F. M.: Reflex epilepsy, behavioral therapy and conditioned reflexes, Springfield, Ill., 1977, Charles C Thomas, Publisher.

Forster, F. M., Klove, H., Petersen, W. G., and Bengzon, A.: Modification of musicogenic epilepsy by extinction techniques, Trans. Am. Neurol. Assoc. **90:**179, 1965.

Forster, F. M., and Booker, H. E.: The epilepsies. In Baker, A. B., editor: Clinical neurology, ed. 4, New York, 1975, Harper & Row, Publishers, Inc.

Jasper, H. H., Ward, A. A., and Pope, A.: Basic mechanisms of the epilepsies, Boston, 1969, Little, Brown & Co., Inc.

Jennett, W. B.: Epilepsy after blunt head injuries, Springfield, Ill., 1962, Charles C Thomas, Publisher.

Penfield, W., and Jasper, H.: Epilepsy and the functional anatomy of the brain, Boston, 1954, Little, Brown & Co., Inc.

Servit, Z.: Reflex mechanisms in the genesis of epilepsy, New York, 1962, Elsevier Publishing Co.

Walker, A. E.: Posttraumatic epilepsy, Springfield, Ill., 1949, Charles C Thomas, Publisher.

Woodbury, D. M., Penry, J. K., and Schmidt, R. P.: Antiepileptic drugs, New York, 1972, Raven Press.

7 Diseases of the basal ganglia—the dyskinesias

The term "basal ganglia" referred originally to the caudate nucleus, putamen, and globus pallidus, but this concept has been broadened to include the red nucleus, substantia nigra, reticular substance, olivary nuclei of the medulla, the locus ceruleus, and by some, even the dentate nucleus.

The various diseases of the basal ganglia manifest themselves clinically by disturbances of movement (dyskinesias).

PARKINSONISM—PARALYSIS AGITANS

The most common disease of the basal ganglia is parkinsonism. The original paper by James Parkinson in 1817 described degenerative types of paralysis agitans. Subsequently it became evident that the same syndrome could be produced by acute encephalitis, arteriosclerosis, neurosyphilis, and manganese or carbon monoxide poisoning, and in more recent years it has been encountered as a toxic manifestation of phenothiazine administration.

The **pathologic lesions** in parkinsonism were necessarily widespread and not restricted to the basal ganglia, or indeed to any one portion of it. Disease processes such as encephalitis, vascular disease, neurosyphilis, or poisoning (for example, with carbon monoxide) could not be expected to observe geographic boundaries within the central nervous system. However, a universal component in cases of parkinsonism studied anatomically was involvement of the substantia nigra.

Biochemical studies, however, opened a vast new area for

exploration and, to date, have been most fruitful in the area of parkinsonism. The demonstrated deficiency in dopamine content and homovanillic acid of the basal ganglia in patients with parkinsonism led to new understandings of the disease process and of treatment. Dopamine is derived from tyrosine through the intermediary action of dihydroxyphenylalanine (dopa) and the enzyme dopa-decarboxylase. Fibers from the substantia nigra to the globus pallidum and putamen are dopaminergic and inhibitory, thus in their normal function preventing excessive outflow from these portions of the basal ganglia. Loss of this inhibitory effect is generally considered to be the cause of the symptomatology.

The **clinical features** of the parkinsonian syndrome consist of hyperkinetic and hypokinetic characteristics. The increased activity (hyperkinetic) is evidenced by a rhythmic tremor, at the rate of four to six per second, which is due to alternate contractions of agonist and antagonist muscles. The **tremor** most commonly affects the hands. Tremor in the hands is frequently predominantly distal—hence the definition of pill rolling. Greater joints, of course, are also involved and, indeed, may be exclusively involved. The lower extremities are often affected by the tremor. Also the muscles of the neck may be afflicted with tremor so that the head is constantly nodding at the same frequency. This affliction of the head is best observed with the patient in profile. With the patient's jaw relaxed and slightly open, the same tremor can often be seen in the jaw. When the mouth is partly open and the jaw relaxed, this same tremor may be seen to involve the tongue. The tremor disappears during sleep, is decreased by active motion of the part, and is increased when the part involved is inactive. Placing the patient in the typical parkinsonian posture also enhances the tremor, as does emotional stress.

Other hyperkinetic features include oculogyric crises, blepharospasms, and restless, almost compulsive, movements. These features occur in parkinsonism due to encephalitis and phenothiazine therapy. **Oculogyric crises** are sudden forceful deviations of the eyes, usually upward but sometimes downward or laterally and persisting for a few seconds to hours. **Blespharospasm** is involuntary, forcible, rapid blinking of the eyes. **Restless, compulsive movements** may be manifested by crossing and uncrossing of the legs, folding and unfolding of the hands, and similar instances of increased activity.

The **hypokinetic features** of parkinsonism are striking. They may be evident long before the tremor appears and, indeed, may be the only manifestations of the syndrome in some patients. The hypokinetic features are characterized by a paucity of motion. When the arms are involved, associated movements are lacking in the arm swing as the patient walks. When sitting down or rising from a chair, the patient does not move his feet prior to changing his position. When he is seated, he will remain motionless for prolonged periods of time, avoiding those frequent small movements that provide comfort. All those movements that are called ''form'' in sports or ''grace'' in dancing are missing in the patient's voluntary actions. Therefore, when bidden in turn, the patient turns en masse rather than the seriatim turning of the head, then the shoulders, and then the pelvic girdle, with the extra little movements of the hands and feet. These are all eschewed, and the body is turned like a statue. Paucity of motion is also evident in the handwriting. Words are written in small, cramped style. (If tremor is present, it is also evident in the handwriting.) Even the speech is affected by paucity of movement. The patient talks with a minimum of inflection, giving a monotonous, weak quality to the sound of the voice. Hypokinesia is evident in the muscles of facial expression, and the patient has a fixed, somewhat austere appearance. Remarkably these patients, when startled, have normal reflex movements. They can catch a falling object involuntarily and do so in a normal fashion, only to resume quickly their previous paucity of motion and tremor.

The **paucity of motion** is present in the gait. The steps become shortened and shuffling. As the disease progresses, the patient's trunk becomes anteflexed so that he leans forward, carrying his arms adducted to the chest and flexed at the elbow and wrist. This is the typical parkinsonian posture. In testing a parkinsonian patient with minimal or no tremor, placing him in this position often will demonstrate an otherwise latent tremor.

A characteristic of hypokinesia is **cogwheel rigidity.** When the involved extremity is alternately flexed and extended, a ratchetlike alternation of movement is elicited. Frequently it is most apparent at the wrist and ankle, but it may be elicited in the neck and, indeed, in the eyes when the patient is asked to follow an object from side to side. Frequently the patient blinks each time the eyes cross the midline. Cogwheeling in the upper extremities can be enhanced by having the patient alternately pat his chest with the hand opposite the one being examined. In the lower extremities it can be demonstrated by having the patient tap the floor with the foot on the side opposite the leg that is being examined for rigidity.

Certain **autonomic changes** are found in patients with parkinsonism, especially of the postencephalitic type. These changes include increased salivation, swelling, and discoloration and coolness of the skin of the extremities. The increased salivation becomes even more troublesome with the development of difficulty in swallowing that is linked to the paucity of movement.

The symptoms in parkinsonism are steadily progressive. Stationary cases (when the disease process has run its course) can occur, expecially in the cases due to toxic states, such as manganese and carbon monoxide poisoning.

In the **treatment** of parkinsonism dopa administration is the mainstay. Levodopa is administered, since it is the precursor of dopamine, and thus the dopamine deficiency in the basal ganglia can be offset. At the present time this requires comparatively large doses, and the oral dose usually is begun at 1 Gm/24 hr in divided doses of four and gradually increased until the desired therapeutic effect is reached, toxic signs appear, or a top dose of 4 to 5 Gm/24 hr is reached. Side effects include gastrointestinal disturbance with nausea and vomiting, dyskinesias of choreic or athetotic type, hypotensive episodes, and rarely, psychosis or blood dyscrasias.

Levodopa is rapidly converted to dopamine in extracerebral tissues. This necessitates the use of large doses and therefore increases the possibility of side effects. Carbidopa inhibits the extracerebral decarboxylation of levodopa and does not cross the blood-brain barrier. The simultaneous administration of levodopa and carbidopa increases the amount of levodopa available in the cerebral tissues and results in lower dosages and fewer side effects. The combination of the two (Sinemet) contains both carbidopa and levodopa in a ratio of 1:10. Care must be taken in transferring patients from levodopa alone to the combination; the levodopa must be discontinued for a short period of time.

The beneficial effects of the dopamine therapies are often dramatic, and previously bedridden patients become ambulatory. The beneficial effects are primarily directed against the hypokinetic features, and the tremor is only slightly decreased. However, with relatively prolonged treatment—six months or more—significant decrease of tremor can occur.

Other medications can also be employed in the treatment of milder cases or cases in which levodopa therapy is contraindicated because of the presence of psychosis, hypotensive states, or cardiac dysrhythmias. The most important of these drugs are the parasympatholytic drugs, including trihexyphenidyl (Artane), benzotropine (Cogentin), procyclidine (Kemadrin), cycrimine (Pagitane), caramiphen (Panparnit), biperiden (Akineton), and ethopropazine (Parsidol). Of these, Artane is the most widely used, being the mainstay of treatment in most patients. When the dosage level of 5 mg/24 hr is reached using the tablets, a 5 mg Artane Sequel may be substituted, providing a more even distribution of medication during the day and still allowing the use of the increased dosage of Artane or of the other parasympatholytic drugs. Toxic symptoms of dizziness and drowsiness are slight and are usually encountered only with higher dosages. Antihistaminic drugs and ampheta-

Table 4
Drugs useful in treating parkinsonism

Action	Preparation	Size of available tablets
Dopamine replacement	Levodopa (Dopar)	100, 250, and 500 mg capsules
Synthetic para-sympatholytic	Carbidopa-levodopa (Sinemet)	10/100 and 25/250
	Biperiden (Akineton)	2 mg tablets
	Trihexyphenidyl (Artane)	2 and 5 mg tablets; 5 mg Artane Sequels
	Benzotropine (Cogentin)	2 mg tablets
	Procyclidine (Kemadrin)	5 mg tablets
	Cycrimine (Pagitane)	1.25 and 2.5 mg tablets
	Caramiphen (Panparnit)	12.5 and 50 mg tablets
	Ethopropazine (Parsidol)	10 and 50 mg tablets
Antihistaminic	Diphenhydramine (Benadryl)	25 mg capsules
	Phenindamine (Thephorin)	25 mg tablets
	Dimenhydrinate (Dramamine)	50 mg tablets
	Promethazine (Phenergan)	12.5 and 25 mg tablets
Stimulant	Amphetamine (Benzedrine)	5 and 10 mg tablets
	Dextroamphetamine (Dexedrine)	5 mg tablets; 5, 10, and 15 mg Spansules
Other	Amantadine (Symmetrel)	100 mg capsules

mines are especially useful in the postencephalitic patients with severe psychomotor retardation. Muscle relaxant drugs play a small role in the control of rigidity. Amantadine (Symmetrel), originally designed as an antiviral agent, has some antiparkinson effect, but this may be temporary.

Medical therapy has considerable effect on the rigidity and hypokinetic factors of parkinsonism but little effect on the tremor. Although medical therapy has considerable effect on the symptoms of parkinsonism, especially the rigidity and hypokinetic elements, the result is not a cure. After a delay of months or even years, the disease continues its relentless course. The progressive loss of nigral cells leads to a decrease in the ability of the substantia nigra to generate dopamine from levodopa. Hence recent attention has focused on the use of dopamine agonists. Of these agents, investigations in progress suggest that bromocriptine may become of value in patients who no longer are responding to levodopa.

Surgical therapy aimed at destruction of the globus pallidus or thalamic nuclei helps certain selected patients.

The parkinsonian syndrome, more or less well developed, may also occur as part of a more serious nervous system disease. Some of these entities may be restricted in distribution, for example, the combination of parkinsonism and dementia seen on Guam among the indigenous Chamorro people. The parkinsonian picture may also be complicated by urinary incontinence and severe autonomic disturbances with marked postural hypotension (Shy-Drager syndrome). Supranuclear ocular palsies may also occur with it (Olszewski syndrome).

ATHETOSIS

The term "athetosis" was derived from the Greek by William Alexander Hammond. It means literally "without a fixed position," thus referring to the constant involuntary movements. Athetosis is a relatively rare condition that can be caused by (1) antenatal malformation (the so-called "état marbré," or status marmoratus, which is a disturbance of myelinization of the caudate nucleus and of the putamen), or (2) more frequently hypoxia, trauma, or infection in the antenatal, perinatal, or immediate postnatal period. Athetosis is often present in patients with cerebral diplegia (cerebral palsy).

The **clinical features** of athetosis seldom are evident at birth, but as the child begins to make purposeful movements, the involuntary movements interfere and become obvious. The involuntary movements are slow, wormlike, muscular contractions involving distal and proximal musculature, producing writhing, somewhat grotesque movements not only of the extremities but also of the trunk and neck and even of the face and vocal apparatus. Therefore in the patients with double (bilateral) athetosis, speech is erratic with sudden forcefulness and alternations in timber. Often it has a nasal quality. The movements are often described as purposeful, since they can be seen to bear some resemblance to purposeful movement.

There is no really successful **treatment** for athetosis. Various surgical procedures have been tried without significant success. The commonly used medications for parkinsonism may be tried.

CHRONIC FAMILIAL CHOREA (HUNTINGTON'S CHOREA)

Familial chorea is a heredodegenerative disease transmitted as a dominant character.

The **pathology** of this disease is a progressive neuronal degeneration of the basal ganglia, particularly of the caudate nucleus and of the cortex of the frontal lobes.

The **clinical picture** generally is not developed until early middle life, usually in the mid-thirties, and is characterized by dyskinesia followed later by mental changes. The dyskinesia consists of quick, jerky involuntary movements, although frequently they have, in addition, a slow component that is sometimes described as choreoathetoid in type. The involuntary movements involve the extremities, trunk, face, and tongue. In the early stages the patients tend to hide these involuntary movements by melding them into a purposeful act, but sooner or later this becomes impossible. The involuntary movements become more frequent and erratic, result in disturbance of gait and dropping of objects and so gradually become more obvious.

The mental changes are chiefly those of deterioration with a progressive organic mental syndrome and, frquently, marked paranoid tendencies.

Treatment is difficult. The disease is steadily progressive, and it is almost invariably necessary eventually to institutionalize the patient because of mental changes. The involuntary movements are difficult to control. Sometimes they can be controlled by the administration of large doses of reserpine, a phenothiazine derivative (Compazine), haloperidol (Haldol), or deanol (Deaner) but without effect on the mental status.

ACUTE CHOREA (SYDENHAM'S CHOREA)

Acute chorea is usually observed in children. It is rare in infants and uncommon in adults, especially as the first attack. This disease is closely related to rheumatic fever. Indeed most neurologists consider it to be a manifestation of rheumatic fever.

The **clinical features** are characterized by the development of sudden, quick, jerky involuntary movements that involve all extremities, the trunk, face, and neck. The movements occur in random fashion without particular pattern or sequence and give rise to facial grimacing and severe, almost flinging movements of the extremities. The severity and frequency of the involuntary movements vary considerably. They may be so severe that the patient is kept in a constant state of activity— hence the old term "St. Vitus' dance." The patients may have numerous bruises from hitting the sides of the bed and other objects during episodes of the uncontrollable movements.

The presence of certain signs helps to confirm the diagnosis of Sydenham's chorea, including (1) the pronator sign (when the arms are held above the head, the hands tend to deviate laterally and pronate); (2) dishing of the hands (when the arms are held extended at the shoulder and the fingers are spread widely, dishing of the hands occurs, that is, flexion at the wrist and hyperextension of the fingers); (3) "milking sign" (with continued hand grasp the patient's fingers alternately grip and relax slightly); and (4) tongue snapping (when the tongue is protruded, it snaps back quickly in almost violent fashion). Patients with Sydenham's chorea may show signs of other widespread neurologic involvement, including pyramidal tract signs. In the patients with more severe disease, mental changes can occur (chorea insaniens). The mental picture is that of restlessness, insomnia, confusion, and delirium. Chorea gravidarum is a recurrence of Sydenham's chorea in the mother at the time of pregnancy or delivery.

Present-day **treatment** consists of complete bed rest, protection, if necessary, against injury by padding the side rails of the bed, and the use of tranquilizing agents, especially prochlorperazine (Compazine), a phenothiazine derivative, in relatively large doses. When rheumatic fever is definitely present, penicillin as well as other measures for the treatment of the disease must be instituted.

HEMICHOREA-HEMIBALLISMUS

Hemichorea is a relatively rare entity, due to lesion sof the contralateral subthalamic nucleus (corpus Luysi). The lesions are most frequently vascular, although neoplasms, including metastatic neoplasms, have been reported to be the etiologic agent. Usually, however, the cause is a small infarct or hemorrhage in this area of the brain. Hemiballismus may follow surgical procedures to alleviate parkinsonism.

Clinically, in view of the nature of the cause, hemichorea generally occurs in older patients and in patients with evidence of cardiovascular cerebral disease. The onset is abrupt. The symptoms consist of wild involuntary movements of the arm and hand or leg, usually both; the trunk and neck also may be affected. The movements are wild and flinging, described as throwing movements (hemiballismus). The severity is such that these patients often lie on the affected side, placing the affected arm under the body or placing the normal leg on top of the affected one to decrease the movements. These movements are disabling. Since these patients often have diminished cardiac reserve, and anxiety is coupled with the increased motor activity, the life of the patient may be threatened by cardiac decompensation.

Since the movements tend to disappear in sleep, the **treatment** includes sedation to give the patient rest. In addition to sedatives, tranquilizing agents such as Compazine and reserpine should be tried. It is often necessary to use surgical procedures to arrest these movements to save the patient's life. Ablations of the motor cortex are relatively simple and in these patients may cause considerable weakness, in addition to relieving the involuntary movements. Since in some patients the hemichorea will disappear in four to seven days after its appearance, it is not necessary to consider surgical procedures immediately unless the patient's general condition is desperate.

HEPATOLENTICULAR DEGENERATION

Hepatolenticular degeneration is a rare familial disease produced by metabolic disturbance, the complete nature of which is not yet clear. There is definitely a deficiency of ceruloplasmin and a decrease of total copper in the plasma, and excess copper is detected in the tissues and urine, together with aminoaciduria. In this disease a defect occurs in the copper-binding mechanism with a failure to bind copper to serum globulins, and about one half of the copper content is bound instead to albumin and thus can be taken up by the proteins of the brain and liver.

The **clinical features** vary from a simple parkinsonian-like manifestation to a more complicated basal ganglia dyskinesia. Involuntary movements in many ways resemble those of patients with Huntington's chorea but are much more forcible. Indeed, these great forcible movements of the upper extremities have been called "Fluegelschlagen," or "wing-beating" movements. The involuntary movements may also be simply parkinsonian in type.

A characteristic feature that, is not always present however, is the lemon-yellowish discoloration of the iris at the limbus, which progresses to a full circular discoloration like a ring around the distal portion of the iris (Kayser-Fleischer ring).

Laboratory studies reveal not only the copper and ceruloplasmin abnormalities but also aminoaciduria and moderate to severe liver function abnormalities (due to cirrhosis).

In **treatment** the antiparkinsonian drugs other than levodopa can be employed in an attempt to alleviate the dyskinesia. This, however, is seldom satisfactory. Treatment with BAL (dimercaprol) and other chelating agents such as penicillamine has been successful in modifying the course of the disease.

SPASMODIC TORTICOLLIS

Spasmodic torticollis is a rare form of dyskinesia characterized by involuntary turning of the head to one side and rotation of the chin upward. This torticollis is not to be confused with the torticollis of the newborn infant (wryneck) due to hemorrhage or trauma to the sternomastoid muscle at parturition. The latter condition is purely local and muscular in origin. Spasmodic torticollis develops later in life and seldom is purely a disorder of the basal ganglia, although cases have been proved to result from an organic disturbance. Many cases, however, are psychogenic in origin. A helpful point of differentiation between the organic and functional spasmodic torticollis is the deviation of the chin upward during the jerky involuntary turning of the head in patients with organic cases. It has been demonstrated that conditioning techniques, using methods of avoidance of feedback, can be employed in the treatment of torticollis. Various medications have proved unsuccessful in most cases.

PIGMENTARY DEGENERATION OF GLOBUS PALLIDUS

Pigmentary degeneration of the globus pallidus and substantia nigra (Hallervorden-Spatz disease) is a rare familial disease occurring in children and characterized by spastic quadriplegia and dysarthria.

SPASTIC PSEUDOSCLEROSIS

Spastic pseudosclerosis (Jakob-Creutzfeldt disease) consists of pyramidal tract signs and tremors, rigidity, dysarthria, akinesia, and almost always mental deterioration. It is caused by degeneration of the cortex, basal ganglia, and spinal cord. This disease occurs in middle or late life and leads to death within a few months or years. It has been successfully transmitted to chimpanzees, thus establishing an infectious etiology for what had been considered a degenerative disease of later life.

KERNICTERUS

Kernicterus is caused by pigmentary staining of the basal ganglia in patients with erythroblastosis fetalis. Kernicterus is usually fatal, although it is possible that institutionalized patients with basal ganglia and cortical diseases have this disorder as at least part of their etiology.

Kernicterus is preventable. Careful serologic studies on the pregnant woman can indicate, by the presence of antibodies, that an incompatibility exists in the blood type, especially the Rh factors, between mother and fetus. Total blood transfusions immediately after birth can prevent the damage to the infant's nervous system.

DYSTONIA MUSCULORUM DEFORMANS

Dystonia musculorum deformans is a severe type of bilateral athetoid disturbance that closely resembles athetosis clinically. However, the disease is degenerative, begins in childhood, and is more marked. The axial musculature is involved to a greater degree in patients with dystonia than in those with athetosis, and dystonia is progressive. It is a rare degenerative disease of unknown etiology.

TARDIVE DYSKINESIA

Tardive dyskinesia consists of involuntary mouthing movements, often accompanied by movement of the tongue. The dyskinesia is bilateral. It is usually the side effect of medications such as the phenothiazines but may occur spontaneously. It occurs more frequently in women and the aged.

GILLES DE LA TOURETTE SYNDROME

The Gilles de la Tourette syndrome occurs in children, begins with involuntary ticlike movements, followed by behavioral changes that include echolalia and coprolalia. This is not definitely a disease of the basal ganglia. However, haloperidol and to a lesser extent phenothiazine are effective therapeutic agents, blocking dopamine receptors in the striatum.

REFERENCES

Diseases of the basal ganglia, Proceedings of the Association meetings held in New York, Dec. 20-21, 1940 and Dec. 5-6, 1975, Assoc. Res. Nerv. & Ment. Dis., Proc. **21:**1-719, 1942; **55:**1-474, 1976.

Calne, D. B.: Developments in the pharmacology and therapeutics of parkinsonism, Ann. Neurol. **1:**111, 1977.

Cooper, I. S.: The neurosurgical alleviation of parkinsonism, Springfield, Ill., 1956, Charles C Thomas, Publisher.

Costa, E., Cote, L. J., and Yahr, M. D.: Biochemistry and pharmacology of the basal ganglia, Proceedings of Second Symposium in New York, 1966, Raven Press.

Denny-Brown, D.: Diseases of the basal ganglia and subthalamic body, New York, 1946, Oxford University Press.

Fields, W. S: Pathogenesis and treatment of parkinsonism, Springfield, Ill., 1958, Charles C Thomas, Publisher.

Gibbs, C. J., Jr., Gadjusek, D. C., Asken, D. M., Alpen, M. P., Bech, E., Daniel, P. M., and Matthews, W. B.: Creutzfeldt-Jakob disease: transmission to the chimpanzee, Science **161:**384, 1968.

Lieberman, A., et al.: Treatment of Parkinson's disease with bromocriptine, N. Engl. J. Med. **295:**1400, 1976.

Onuaguluchi, G.: Parkinsonism, London, 1964, Butterworth & Co. (Publishers), Ltd.

Richmond, J., Rosenoer, V. M., Tompsett, S. L., Draper, I., and Simpson, J. A.: Hepato-lenticular disease (Wilson's disease) treated by penicillamine, Brain **87:**619, 1964.

Yahr, M. D., Duvoisin, R. C., Schear, M. J., Barrett, R. E., and Hoehn, M. M.: Treatment of parkinsonism with levodopa, Arch. Neurol. **21:**343, 1969.

8 Multiple sclerosis and other demyelinizing diseases

MULTIPLE SCLEROSIS

Multiple sclerosis is a particularly vexing problem in neurology because it is a disease unlike that of any other system of the body. This disease has an overall incidence of between 5 and 75 per 100,000. Although it is slightly more common in women than in men, the difference is not significant. Two thirds of the cases occur in persons between the ages of 20 and 40 years. Rarely is multiple sclerosis seen in patients in the first decade of life and then only at the very end of that decade.

The fundamental **pathology** of multiple sclerosis has three characteristics: demyelination, partial destruction of the axis cylinders, and gliosis. The demyelination is geographic and sharp in outline. The axis cylinders in the demyelinized areas are partially destroyed, although an appreciable number of axis cylinders are left in the plaque. In the course of time, astrocytes form a gliotic scar in the area of demyelination. These three features—demyelination, partial destruction of axis cylinders, and gliosis—comprise the pathology of the individual lesion in patients with multiple sclerosis. Early incomplete lesions are probably reversible. The characteristics of the lesions, in addition to the three major features, are that in a given case they are randomly distributed in the central nervous system and vary in age. In the same patient can be found acute lesions with minimal or early gliosis, old lesions with dense scarring, and lesions intermediate in age.

The lesions of multiple sclerosis are scattered "in time and place"; that is, they not only vary in age but also in location. There is no particular rhyme or reason to the distribution. The lesions involve the entire central nervous system—cerebrum, brain stem, cerebellum, spinal cord, and the optic nerve and its tract (which are actually prolongations of the central nervous sytem). Peripheral nerves, however, are seldom if ever primarily involved. The lesions occur only in the white matter. They may involve gray matter almost by accident, that is, by contiguity, but the lesions are not primarily found in gray matter. Although there is no particular reason for the location of the lesions, they tend to occur particularly in the periventricular areas.

The **etiology** in this disease remains obscure. A number of theories have been evolved and tested over a period of years, but none of these has been proved or has adequately explained the cause of this disease. The theory of infection has been promulgated on several occasions, and various organisms, including spirochetes, have been implicated. These older concepts have been disproved. At the present time it is conceivable that multiple sclerosis is caused by a slow virus, perhaps related to or identical with the measles virus. Vascular etiology has been suspected, particularly because many of the lesions tend to occur about veins, especially in the early phases of the disease. However, conclusive evidence has not been forthcoming that its origin is based on occlusion or spasm of vessels. Allergy and deficiency have been involved, but these too have failed to explain in toto the etiology of this disease. Many studies suggest that multiple sclerosis is an autoimmune disease.

The cardinal **clinical features** of multiple sclerosis are multiple signs and symptoms of nervous system involvement with remissions and exacerbations. The signs and symptoms indicate disseminated involvement of the nervous system.

Certain **signs and symptoms** are **commonly seen** in patients with multiple sclerosis. Often the first symptoms of multiple sclerosis are so slight that the patient does not seek a physician. Therefore the account of these early symptoms is obtained only in retrospect and after the onset of a more major portion of the illness. Early signs in this category are transient paresthesias of the extremities, transient diplopia lasting for a few minutes to several days, transient blurring of vision lasting for a few hours to a day or so, a short period of clumsiness in the use of the extremities or mild to moderate weakness of one extremity, and slight bouts of vertigo. Frequently in these early stages symptoms are considered to be of functional origin. A mild, often slight sign described by Lhermitte is a sensory response to flexion of the chin on the chest. The sensory response is a vibratory tingling, or electrical feeling, that may go up and down the spine or across the shoulders or may even be felt in the lower extremities.

The more severe signs of multiple sclerosis are (1) marked cerebellar signs (for example, disturbances of gait, incoordination in the use of the extremities, and speech disturbances such as scanning speech); (2) pyramidal tract signs (for example, significant weakness with or without spasticity and signs such as hyperreflexia, Hoffmann's sign of the fingers, Babinski and Chaddock toe signs, and clonus in the lower extremities); (3) visual disturbances, with the development of a frank optic atrophy and impaired acuity that cannot be corrected by refraction, and the occurrence of visual scotomas; (4) signs due to the involvement of the nuclei of the extraocular muscles or of the pathways between these nuclei including diplopia and nystagmus that may be permanent; (5) bladder disturbances (such as urinary retention or incontinence); and (6) evidence of lesions in the white matter of the frontal lobe that produce personality changes, frequently with a facetiousness and a disregard for the seriousness of the patient's illness. The latter is not always present, however. Sometimes patients, instead, become irritable and even paranoid. These more severe signs may be insidious in onset and gradual, but not infrequently they are abrupt and almost apoplectic. Therefore the patient may present with an acute transverse myelitis or acute hemiplegia.

Certain **signs and symptoms** are extremely **uncommon** in patients with multiple sclerosis. When these occur, one should
suspect that some other disease entity is the cause of the varied
symptomatology. These uncommon evidences are homonymous hemianopsia, aphasia, convulsive seizures, severe pain
syndromes, and signs of anterior horn cell disease. Any of
these symptoms can occur in patients with multiple sclerosis,
but since they are atypical, they warrant a careful evaluation to
ascertain that the patient does not have another disease that
can give evidence of such dissemination.

Diagnostic studies in multiple sclerosis include special visual
studies and examination of the spinal fluid, and it appears that
special studies of circulating lymphocytes may be of diagnostic
value in the future. The visual examinations are of special
value in patients with perplexing neurologic signs and
symptoms of other portions of the central nervous system, for
example, of the spinal cord, but no history of visual complaints. Demonstration in these patients of involvement of the
optic nerve or tract is evidence of disseminated nervous system involvement. Careful plotting of the visual fields with
tangent screen or by Goldmann perimetry may show a
scotoma. Even more definitive is the use of visual evoked potentials to demonstrate the presence of lesions especially
asymptomatic lesions, of the visual system. In a high percentage of patients there are abnormalities of the spinal fluid, including a slight degree of pleocytosis, a moderate increase in
the amount of protein, changes in the colloidal gold reaction,
and an elevated gamma globulin content. The pleocytosis is
mild. Therefore if more than ten cells are present, one may
suspect that the diagnosis is incorrect. The total protein content is seldom over 100 mg/100 ml. The study of circulating
lymphocytes is still in the experimental stage. This is concerned with the mobility of lymphocytes as seen in the
cytopherometer and with fluorescence studies involving
specific viruses.

Individual **prognosis** of multiple sclerosis is difficult. In 10%
of patients the course is a steady progression, whereas in 90%

relapses and remissions occur. Even in the 10%, however, if one follows their condition carefully, there are minor remissions and exacerbations, but the course is nevertheless endlessly progressive. It is impossible to predict the recurrence of exacerbations in this disease, since these vary from four or five a year to one in twenty years in the individual patient. The exacerbations follow no predictable pattern. The average life expectancy after the onset of the disease is twenty-seven years. Although the disease may not materially decrease the life expectancy, it certainly decreases life efficiency.

Treatment of multiple sclerosis can be divided into general supportive, specific, and symptomatic categories.

General supportive therapy includes careful maintenance of nutrition and avoidance of trauma whenever possible. Young people with this disease should be interdicted from contact sports. Unnecessary surgical procedures should not be performed. However, when surgery is necessary, care should be taken in the choice of anesthetics. It is wise to avoid anesthetics that are fat solvents, for example, ether, and, of course, spinal anesthesia should not be used. Pregnancy does not seem to have a deleterious effect on the course of multiple sclerosis, despite some of the earlier statistical studies on this subject.

At present, since the etiology is obscure, there is no **specific therapy** aimed at the treatment of the disease process. Numerous attempts at specific therapy have been made. None has yet proved successful. The most recent specific or quasi-specific therapeutic attempt has been the use of ACTH. The results of this therapy are equivocal in general, although there is sufficient evidence to warrant its use in acute episodes of multiple sclerosis.

Symptomatic therapy is largely concerned with the control of the symptoms that the patient has developed. In the treatment of weakness and spasticity, the most important factor is the use of medicine and rehabilitative techniques aimed at producing the maximum function and also at maintaining the spirits of the patient. Drugs aimed at muscle relaxation, such as diazepam (Valium), are helpful in reducing spasticity, but the dosage must be carefully titrated to avoid increasing muscular weakness. The decrease in visual acuity cannot be aided by refraction. Little success is to be expected in the treatment of visual disturbances. If the diplopia is permanent, patching of one eye may be required and should be done alternately to avoid weakening the vision of either eye. Bladder disturbances may be particularly difficult to manage. In the milder phases of urinary retention, administration of bethanechol (Urecholine) may aid in reducing retention. In patients with urinary frequency, propantheline (Pro-banthine) will sometimes decrease the urgency and frequency. In patients with more severe disturbances of the bladder, it is important to maintain an indwelling catheter and various drainage procedures. Tidal drainage, when used carefully and systematically, will produce an improvement in bladder function in some cases so that catheterization may be discontinued.

DIFFUSE SCLEROSIS

Much less common in incidence are the diseases grouped together under the term "diffuse sclerosis." The most common of these is **encephalitis periaxialis diffusa (Schilder's disease).**

Pathologically, Schilder's disease is a demyelination of both hemispheres, beginning usually in the white matter of the occipital lobe and extending forward. Demyelination is marked. The special characteristic is the preservation of the subcortical U fibers.

Clinically, Schilder's disease affects young children, especially boys. It occurs in childhood, usually before the age of puberty. The onset may be abrupt, and the course is steady and relentless. Death generally occurs within several months, although the course may extend as long as a year or two. The clinical picture is characterized by blindness that is cerebral in type, since there is no involvement of the optic nerve. The blindness is followed by deafness and mental deterioration, bilateral spasticity, and seizures.

A number of rare forms of diffuse sclerosis (which are usually named for the author who first described them) include **encephalitis periaxialis concentrica (Balo's disease)** and **chronic infantile cerebral**

sclerosis (Merzbacher-Pelizaeus disease), as well as the forms described by **Krabbe** and by **Scholz.**

NEUROMYELITIS OPTICA (DEVIC'S DISEASE)

Neuromyelitis optica is probably not a spearate disease but the concurrence of optic neuritis or retrobulbar neuritis and transverse myelitis within a relatively short period of time. Most authors believe that patients with these syndromes are really multiple sclerosis patients whose lesions happen to give rise to this constellation of symptoms and signs.

ACUTE DISSEMINATED ENCEPHALOMYELITIS

Acute disseminated encephalomyelitis is also a questionable entity and, in essence, is an acute episode of rather severe multiple sclerosis with involvement of many parts of the nervous system simultaneously. It may also be confused with an acute encephalomyelitis of the perivenous type (p. 143) due to a particular etiology.

REFERENCES

Bauer, H. J., and Firnhaber, W.: Prognostic criteria in multiple sclerosis, Ann. N. Y. Acad. Sci. **122:**542, 1965.
Ellenberger, C., Jr., and Zeigler, S. B.; Visual evoked potentials and quantitative perimetry in multiple sclerosis, Ann. Neurol. **1:**561, 1977.
McAlpine, D., Compston, N. D., and Lumsden, C. D.: Multiple sclerosis, London, 1955, E. & S. Livingstone, Ltd.
McAlpine, D., Lumsden, C. E., and Acheson, E. O.: Multiple sclerosis: a reappraisal, Baltimore, 1972, Williams & Wilkins Co.
Multiple sclerosis and the demyelinating diseases, Proceedings of the Association meeting held in New York, Dec. 10-11, 1948, Assoc. Res. Nerv. & Ment. Dis., Proc. **28:**1-675, 1950.
Rose, A. S., and Pearson, C. M.: Mechanics of demyelination, New York, 1963, McGraw-Hill Book Co.
Schumacher, G. A.: Symposium on multiple sclerosis and demyelinationg diseases, Am. J. Med. **12:**499, 1952.
Schumacher, G. A.: Multiple sclerosis and other demyelinating diseases. In Forster, F. M., editor: Modern therapy in neurology, St. Louis, 1957, The C. V. Mosby Co.
Symposium on disseminated sclerosis, Proc. Roy. Soc. Med. **54:**1, 1961.

9 Tumors of the central nervous system

Tumors occur in the central nervous system in a much higher incidence than is usually appreciated. As many as 9% of all tumors occur in the central nervous system. In a large autopsy series of central nervous system tumors, 80% occurred in the brain and 20% in the spinal cord.

BRAIN TUMORS
Primary brain tumors

Pathologically, primary brain tumors may be of the glioma series and originate in neural tissue or may arise from other intracranial structures, such as the meninges, blood vessels, sheaths of the cranial nerves, and pituitary gland. The **gliomas,** the most important of the primary tumors, comprise 45% of all brain tumors.

One third of the gliomas are of the type called **glioblastoma multiforme.** This type is highly malignant and characterized by numerous mitotic figures, areas of necrosis, changes in the structure of the blood vessels within the tumor, and a highly variegated type of cell. They occur in persons in the middle to older age groups, almost exclusively in the cerebral hemispheres and have a tendency to cross the midline by invasion of the corpus callosum. As a rule the clinical course is short and seldom lasts longer than twelve to eighteen months.

Astrocytomas also comprise one third of the glioma series. These are much less malignant tumors and are derived from astrocytes. The cell division is usually amitotic rather than mitotic. These tumors are not encapsulated, and the boundary between normal tissue and tumor is difficult to determine. Astrocytomas occur in cerebral hemispheres, brain stem, cerebellum, and spinal cord. In the cerebrum and cerebellum they are often cystic.

Medulloblastomas are highly malignant tumors arising from cell rests in the medullary vellum of the fourth ventricle. They are characterized by primitive cells with numerous mitotic figures. The tumors are invasive and, indeed, may extend into the brain stem by way of the cerebellar peduncles. By metastasis in the subarachnoid space they may cause a secondary tumor enwrapping the spinal cord. This type of tumor occurs almost exclusively in children.

Ependymomas arise from ependymal cells. These tumors occur in the cerebral hemisphere, in the floor of the fourth ventricle (in infants and young children), and in the spinal cord (in older patients). They are the most common intramedullary spinal cord tumors.

Oligodendrogliomas, which occur in the cerebral hemispheres and less commonly in the brain stem and spinal cord, are tumors derived from the oligodendroglia cells. Like the astrocytomas they are relatively mature and slow-growing tumors.

Tumors of the meninges are most commonly **meningiomas** and comprise fibroblastic elements and arachnoidal cell types. In the more mature types of meningiomas, the cells occur in whirls around flecks of calcium deposited in degenerated cells (so-called psammoma bodies). Meningiomas vary in the amount of fibroblastic and endothelial tissue in the individual tumor. They may be very vascular; indeed, in rare instances they may resemble histologically a hemangioblastoma. Meningiomas are encapsulated, slow-growing, and frequently of large size. There is, however, a small, thin, flat tumor called *meningiome en plaque*. Very rarely the tumor may undergo malignant changes. Meningiomas occur intracranially over the vertex, along the falx, and at the base of the skull, in the olfactory groove, about the sella, and occasionally in the posterior fossa; they also occur in the spinal canal.

Tumors can arise from blood vessels. The true **hemangioma** is not really a neoplasm but an anomaly of numerous blood vessels normal and abnormal, laid down in a particular area of the brain. The **hemangioblastoma,** however, is a tumor derived from blood vessel tissue and is made up of endothelial cells and some fibroblastic cells. Hemangioblastomas are most common in the cerebellum and are uncommon in the cerebral hemispheres. These tumors are often associated with hemangiomas of the retina (von Hippel-Lindau disease) and with polycythemia.

Pinealomas, because of their location, compress the quadrigeminal plate and the aqueduct of Sylvius. Clinically they produce greatly increased intracranial pressure and early in the course cause paralysis of upward ocular gaze (Parinaud's sign). Occasionally a pinealoma is aberrant and occurs elsewhere, particularly in the hypothalamus.

Tumors within the cerebral ventricle are uncommon. In early childhood ependymomas may occur in the fourth ventricle. Later in life colloid cysts occur in the lateral or third ventricles. Papillomas and papillocarcinoma can arise from the choroid plexus. Intraventricular tumors produce as their chief sign evidence of increased intracranial pressure. A characteristic of the benign tumor that serves as a ball valve is severe headache altered by position.

The **adenomas of the pituitary gland** are differentiated by their staining characteristics. Basophilic adenomas, the cells of which take up a basophilic dye and often have small lacunae within them, are small tumors that do not expand the sella, do not extend from the sella into the cranial vault, and therefore do not involve the adjacent nervous tissue. These tumors may produce hyperadrenalism (Cushing's syndrome) but do not produce neurologic changes, since they remain intrasellar. In general, the most common cause of Cushing's syndrome now is the result of the use of adrenocorticosteroid therapy for the control of another disease process. The most common pathologic cause of Cushing's syndrome is disease of the adrenal glands, rather than pituitary disease.

Chromophobic and eosinophilic adenomas, however, increase sufficiently in size to expand the sella and may extrude from the sella into the intracranial cavity. There they involve nervous tissue, particularly the optic nerves, and may impair the cerebral blood supply by involving the internal carotid arteries. The chromophobic adenomas give rise to the syndrome of pituitary insufficiency. Eosinophilic adenomas produce gigantism when they occur before the fusion of the epiphysis. If they occur after this time, they produce acromegaly.

Tumors of the cranial nerves arise from the sheaths of the nerves and are fibroblastic tumors called neuromas, neurinomas, or perineural fibroblastomas. They are most common on the eighth cranial nerve, may also occur on the fifth cranial nerve, and less frequently are located on the other lower cranial nerves.

Tumors of the optic nerves are gliomas rather than neurinomas because the optic nerve is really an extension of the brain and is not a nerve in the true sense, since it has no perineural, epineural, or endoneural components. Tumors of the optic nerves therefore are astrocytomas or oligodendrogliomas and are true gliomas. Tumors of the optic nerves and neurinomas of the cranial and spinal nerves, as well as meningiomas, occur in association with von Recklinghausen's disease.

Cystic tumors occur in the **suprasellar region.** The synonyms for these are craniopharyngioma, Rathke's pouch tumor, hypophyseal stalk tumor, adamantinoma, and ameloblastoma. These are tumors of congenital origin caused by cell rests from the primitive nasopharynx. These cells come to lie about the hypophyseal stalk. When they undertake neoplastic change, they produce a tumor, usually suprasellar and without distortion of the sella. The tumors contain calcium that is readily demonstrated radiologically. They are largely cystic and contain cholesterol crystals. The capsule is made up of fibrous tissue and epithelium, varying from squamous through the columnar type.

Metastatic tumors to brain

Metastatic tumors to the brain are of increasing importance. These may be carcinomatous or sarcomatous, or they may arise from malignant melanomas; carcinomas are by far the most common. The most frequent sites of origin for these metastases to the brain are the lung and the breast. Carcinomas of the thyroid and the adrenals are less common than the preceding type but have in themselves a high incidence of metastasis to the brain. Metastatic tumors, whether carcinomatous, sarcomatous, or due to melanomas, may be single or multiple solitary tumors within the substance of the brain or may primarily involve the meninges, either the leptomeninges or the dura. When the leptomeninges are invaded, the tumor spreads through the meningeal spaces, crowds into the substance of the brain about the perivascular spaces, and causes numerous small lesions in the parenchyma as well. At the level of the brain stem, invasion into the brain substance may also occur along cranial nerves. Metastases over the dura are usually large fulminating masses, which may invade the bone of the cranial vault.

Clinical signs

The famous triad of brain tumor symptoms, fortunately, is now rarely seen. This triad, consisting of headache, papilledema, and projectile vomiting, is due to a great increase in intracranial pressure. In modern times it is rare indeed for a brain tumor not to be diagnosed long before the development of the full triad.

The so-called **general symptoms** of brain tumor are the result of increased intracranial pressure. The severe headache, occurring well into the course of development of brain tumor, has no localizing value. Generalized seizures occurring in a patient with a brain tumor may not present any clinical evidence of localizing value, except, of course, that they suggest the cerebrum rather than other parts of the brain as the locus for the tumor. Mental changes occur in patients with brain tumors, either because of direct involvement of the frontal lobe or because of increased intracranial pressure. In either event the behavioral symptoms are those of the organic brain syndrome—memory defect, especially recent impaired judgment, impaired arithmetic ability, and change in affect. When this organic mental syndrome occurs after the development of papilledema and increased pressure, it is of no localizing significance. However, if the syndrome developed prior to the intracranial hypertension, a frontal lobe lesion is suspected.

The **focal signs and symptoms** of brain tumors depend on the location of the lesion. The most important characteristic of the signs and symptoms of the brain tumor is that of progression, which indicates a growth and expansion of the tumor. A weakness of the fingers spreading to the wrist, elbow, shoulder, and then the face obviously points to a tumor involving the motor cortex. Mild aphasia, progressing gradually to an increasing degree of language impairment, and visual field defects changing from quadrantic to hemianoptic are obvious signs indicating an expanding cerebral lesion. It is likewise important to recognize a progressive seizure pattern change that cannot be attributed to medication, since this, too, is an indication of an expanding lesion. Indeed, the appearance of seizures after the age of 20 years and certainly after 30 years arouses suspicion of the presence of brain tumor unless the seizures are adequately explained on another basis.

Certain **signs and symptoms** have **limited value** for localization and may even be misleading. The most frequent of these is a partial involvement of the abducens nerve on one side. This can be due to compression of the sixth cranial nerve by the brain stem and is secondary to the increased intracranial pressure. A similar pseudolocalization may occur with pupillary changes and third nerve signs when the uncus herniates and compresses the third nerve. The organic mental syndrome, as noted previously, may be due to increased intracranial pressure, since a posterior fossa tumor can compress the aqueduct producing internal hydrocephalus and frontal lobe damage. A bilateral increase of deep tendon reflexes and plantar signs can occur in a patient with a rapidly growing cerebellar lesion that compresses the pyramidal tracts against the base of the occiput. The appearance of cerebellar signs from cerebral lesions may at times lead to some confusion. A frontal lesion may produce contralateral cerebellar signs by involvement of frontopontocerebellar pathways. Frontal lobe cerebellar signs, however, are not nearly as significant as those which occur in patients with cerebellar lesions.

The **most important tumors of the cerebral hemispheres** are glioblastomas multiforme, astrocytomas, meningiomas, and metastatic tumors. The clinical course is usually short—less than a year in duration—in patients with glioblastoma multiforme or metastatic tumors, whereas in those with astrocytomas and particularly with meningiomas, the clinical course may extend over many years.

Tumors of the cerebellum occur predominantly in children. Medulloblastomas and astrocytomas comprise the majority of them, and hemangioblastomas are rare. The clinical course in patients with medulloblastomas is very acute, whereas that in patients with astrocytomas is usually of longer duration (over a year). The cerebellar astrocytomas are often cystic, and the prognosis is obviously much better in patients with astrocytoma than in those with medulloblastoma.

Tumors of the brain stem are characterized by the progressive destruction of the cranial nerves and their nuclei and long tracts. These tumors occur mostly in children and young adults and are astrocytomas, occasionally oligodendrogliomas, and sometimes less common types such as the spongioblastoma polare.

Tumors of the cranial nerves most commonly involve the eighth cranial nerve. The slowly progressive clinical features include tinnitus, deafness, bouts of vertigo, mild cerebellar signs, involvement of the seventh and fifth cranial nerves on the same side, and signs of cerebellar and pyramidal tract involvement. These are slow-growing tumors occurring in persons in the middle or older age groups and are almost invariably accompanied by a high total protein content in the spinal fluid. They are usually unilateral, but in patients with von Recklinghausen's disease they may be bilateral. Other lesions in the lateral recess or the cerebellar pontine angle may present the same picture. These include meningiomas, aberrant gliomas, hemangiomas, and parasitic infestations, especially cysticercosis.

The **suprasellar cysts,** or craniopharyngiomas, are more common in children and young adults, although they may occur at any age. The clinical manifestations include signs of pressure, including headache, involvement of the optic tracts or nerves, leading to bilateral blindness, optic atrophy, and hypopituitarism.

Diagnostic studies

The diagnostic studies employed in the analysis of a patient in whom brain tumor is suspected include a group of studies that are in themselves not dangerous. Unless there is reason for emergency, these should always be carried out first. This group of studies includes the examination and charting of visual fields, electroencephalography, audiometric and caloric testing when indicated, and radiographic and radioisotopic study.

Visual field studies are important in all patients with suspected tumors of the cerebral hemispheres and of the perichiasmal region. It is important that the visual fields be charted accurately on a perimeter or, preferably, a tangent screen for the purpose of future comparison for changes in the conformation of the fields.

Electroencephalography may demonstrate a slow wave focus with or without a convulsive component in the suspected part of the cerebrum. When there is a significant increase of intracranial pressure, however, the electroencephalogram becomes somewhat difficult to interpret, and it is possible to have false localizing electroencephalographic changes.

Audiometric and caloric tests are of value only in the establishment of function of both components of the acoustic nerve. However, in any patient with suspected brain stem or cranial nerve tumor, these should be recorded for future reference if necessary.

Radiographic studies are probably the most important of these preliminary and nonhazardous studies. It is important in each patient that a chest film be requested as well as studies of the skull. Carcinoma of the lung may metastasize very early to the brain, and the presenting clinical evidence can be that of a brain tumor. The skull film should include anteroposterior, posteroanterior, and right and left lateral films. In patients with brain stem tumors or cranial nerve tumors, the special views of the base of the skull and of the foramina, particularly the internal acoustic meatus, should be sought. When the optic nerve is involved, special views of the optic foramina are important. Points of interest in the radiographic studies are the signs of increased intracranial pressure (demineralization of the clinoids of the sella and hammered silver markings, significant only past the age of 14 years), evidence of bone destruction and erosion by a tumor, abnormal calcification (occurring most frequently in patients with meningiomas, astrocytomas, oligodendrogliomas, and suprasellar cysts), and displacement of normally calcified structures such as the pineal gland or the normally calcified glomus. Minor displacements of the calcified glomus, however, are difficult to interpret, since the glomera may lie in different levels on the two sides.

The CT, or CAT, scan, especially when carried out with the injection of a contrast material, is a safe and highly productive method of testing for the presence of brain tumors. Radioisotope scanning is also of value and should be considered as additive to the CT scan. Whereas in many laboratories radioactive iodine-tagged albumen is the tracer substance of choice when lesions at the base of the skull or over temporal regions are suspected, other agents such as radioactive mercury are preferable, since the density of this is not increased in muscle tissue. Technetium-99 has come into wide usage. This isotope is rapidly assimilated and the test results are readily obtained.

The examination of the cerebrospinal fluid and contrast radiographic studies carry with them considerable hazard, and these studies should not be undertaken unless it is possible to proceed with neurosurgical intervention in the event of emergency. The examination of the spinal fluid is most useful for the demonstration of increased intracranial pressure and elevation of total protein content. The cell count may be elevated; rarely the cells may be found to be neoplastic when stained.

Air contrast studies may be carried out by the lumbar route (pneumoencephalogram) or neurosurgically by the ventricular route (ventriculogram). In patients with increased intracranial pressure or in a patient with a suspected tumor in the posterior fossa, pneumoencephalography by the lumbar route is hazardous, and ventriculography is to be preferred.

Arteriography plays a definite role in the analysis of the brain tumor patient. This study not only may show the site but also give a clue as to the nature of the tumor. The site is indicated by the displacement of vessels, for example, the anterior cerebral artery displaced across the midline or the middle cerebral elevated or depressed. The nature of the tumor may be indicated by a "tumor stain" that suggests a particular type of tumor, such as meningioma or glioblastoma multiforme.

Treatment

The obvious treatment of brain tumors is surgical. There is no positive way to make a histologic diagnosis short of surgery. Therefore every patient is entitled to be explored and have the tumor removed if feasible, even when clinically the course is one to suggest a malignant tumor, unless it is definitely metastatic.

Radiotherapy is useful in certain types of tumors, particularly those which are more malignant, such as glioblastoma multiforme and medulloblastoma, and in certain metastatic tumors. Radiotherapy, particularly in the medulloblastomas, must be vigorous; indeed, the neuraxis should be treated with radiotherapy because of possible seeding from the original tumor into the spinal axis.

Chemotherapy of primary brain tumors has not yet proved successful.

TUMORS OF THE SPINAL CANAL

Pathologically, tumors of the spinal canal may be primary or secondary in origin and either intramedullary or extramedullary, that is, within or without the substance of the spinal cord, in which case they may be either subdural or extradural. **Primary extradural tumors** are meningiomas or neurinomas (perineural fibroblastomas). These types, described previously, grow slowly within the spinal canal, gradually compressing the spinal cord. A rare type of primary extramedullary cord tumor (chordoma) arises from remnants of the notochord, usually in the sacral region. Unlike the meningioma and perineural fibroblastoma, this tumor is malignant.

Metastatic carcinoma is generally extramedullary and rarely intramedullary. Carcinomas arise most commonly from the prostate, breast, and thyroid, metastasize to the substance of the vertebral bodies, and by extension may invade the spinal canal. Their symptoms are caused by compression and by embarrassment of the blood supply of the cord.

Ependymomas are the most common **intramedullary spinal cord tumors.** These are relatively slow growing and often encapsulated. Intramedullary cord tumors are less commonly astrocytomas in type.

Clinical signs

The earliest clinical sign of a spinal cord tumor, particularly if it is extramedullary, is pain. This may begin as vertebral pain and then progress to a root disturbance. It is usually worse at night when the patient is in a recumbent position. It is aggravated by coughing, sneezing, or straining and is followed by evidence of embarrassment of tract function in the cord with weakness, pyramidal tract signs, impairment of bladder control, and sensory loss.

Differentiation between extramedullary and intramedullary

tumors is often difficult, if not impossible, on the basis of clinical findings. However, the early appearance of root pain, the beginning of sensory loss such as saddle anesthesia, and the spread of the anesthetic level upward are more indicative of extramedullary than of intramedullary locations.

Diagnostic studies

The most important laboratory studies in patients with spinal cord tumors are the cerebrospinal fluid and radiologic studies. The cerebrospinal fluid studies may indicate a complete cord block with the spinal fluid presenting the formula of low initial pressure, xanthochromic fluid, increased cells, and elevated total protein. This occurs only when there has been a complete block for some time. More commonly the dynamics are still free, protein is moderately elevated, and the fluid has a slight xanthochromic tinge.

Radiologic studies of the spine may reveal destruction of the vertebral processes, particularly in patients with malignant cord tumors. No indication of the neoplasm may be present with the routine spinal radiographs, particularly in patients with intramedullary tumors. Myelography usually reveals an encroachment on the spinal canal. Indeed, by the nature of the encroachment, the differentiation of extramedullary as opposed to intramedullary tumor may be made by the distribution of oil. The presence of a meniscus or "capping" suggests an extramedullary lesion, whereas widening of the cord shadow indicates an intramedullary process.

Treatment

The treatment of spinal cord tumors is surgical. These patients present emergencies, since once the patient has become paraplegic, little is to be gained by exploration. Early diagnosis and rapid surgical treatment is of the greatest importance. There is a possibility of precipitating the patient into difficulties by spinal fluid examination or myelography when the clinical signs are those of a partial transection of the cord. These pro-

cedures therefore should be carried out when one is prepared
for early exploration if necessary. Radiation therapy is of value
only in patients with malignancies. Chemotherapy is useful
only in patients with those malignancies whose parent cells are
amenable to chemotherapy. In metastatic tumors from the
prostate or breast, the proper hormonal therapy, either surgical or medical, is indicated to hold in abeyance the recurrence
of the secondary tumor.

REFERENCES

Bailey, P.: Intracranial tumors, Springfield, Ill., 1933, Charles C Thomas, Pub-
lisher.
Bailey, P., Buchanan, D. N., and Bucy, P. C.: Intracranial tumors of infancy
and childhood, Chicago, 1939, University of Chicago Press.
Pack, G. T., and Ariel, I. M.: Tumors of the nervous system. In Pack, G. T.,
and Ariel, I. M., editors: Treatment of cancer and allied diseases, Vol. 2,
New York, 1962, Paul B. Hoeber, Inc., Medical Book Department of Harper
& Row, Publishers, Inc.
Rand, R. W., and Rand, C. W.: Intraspinal tumors of childhood, Springfield,
Ill., 1960, Charles C Thomas, Publisher.
Russell, D. S., and Rubinstein, L. J.: Pathology of tumors of the nervous sys-
tem, Baltimore, 1977, The Williams & Wilkins Co.
Sayre, G. P.: The system of grading gliomas, Acta Neurochir. (Wien.) supp.
10, 1964.
Zulch, J. K.: Brain tumors: their biology and pathology, New York, 1965,
Springer Publishing Co., Inc.

10 Infections of the nervous system

MENINGITIS

Anatomically there are two layers of meninges, the more external and thicker dura mater, which adheres to the skull, and the thinner pia-arachnoid, which is closely applied to the brain. Inflammation involving the dura is called pachymeningitis, and inflammation involving the pia-arachnoid is properly called leptomeningitis. Since pachymeningitis is rare, the term "meningitis" in common usage refers to leptomeningitis. Pachymeningitis or leptomengitis may be acute or chronic. In either state leptomeningitis is far more common than pachymeningitis. Pachymeningitis may be either spinal or cranial, whereas leptomeningitis is seldom completely limited to either spinal or cranial areas.

Acute (purulent) leptomeningitis

Almost all known organisms, whether pathogenic or nonpathogenic, have at some time been indicted as a cause of purulent meningitis. However, the most common causative organisms of purulent meningitis are the meningococcus, pneumococcus, influenza bacillus, *Streptococcus,* and *Staphylococcus.* In the newborn infant the coliform organisms *(Escherichia coli)* are an important cause of meningitis. Of all these organisms the meningococcus is usually considered to induce a primary type of meningitis, whereas the others cause meningitis secondary to some other focus of inflammation. Meningococcal meningitis results from seeding of organisms in the leptomeninges early in the course of meningococcal bacteremia.

The other forms of meningitis are secondary to extracerebral disease, such as paranasal sinus, middle ear, and pulmonary infections.

The gross **pathology** of purulent meningitis gives rise to swelling of the brain, with flattening of convolutions and obscuring of the normal gross architecture by the presence of pus. This is most severe over the vertex of the brain and is usually thinner at the base. In patients with meningococcal meningitis the exudate is diffused but is most concentrated anteriorly over the lateral surfaces of the hemispheres. In patients with the other purulent meningitides, the exudate is often thicker and may even have the consistency of a heavy plastic several millimeters thick, which completely obscures the architectural markings of the brain. This exudate is often patchy, and the location of the patchiness depends on the focus from which the meningitis developed, for example, over the right frontal area of the brain when due to right frontal sinusitis.

On histologic examination of patients in the acute stages of meningitis, the leptomeninges are grossly distended and filled with polymorphonuclear cells, organisms, and debris. In patients in the later stages, fibrin has been laid down, and there is a gradual change from polymorphonuclear cells to phagocytes and lymphocytes. If the exudate has been heavy, there is a corresponding degree of fibrosis. Usually the pia-glial barrier is not violated, and the leptomeninges are clearly distinguished from the cerebral tissue. Later, when there is a significant degree of fibrosis, however, there may be matting down of the leptomeninges against the cortex.

The **clinical signs** of acute meningitis are divisible into those of febrile diseases in general and those of meningitis specifically. The general signs of febrile disease are fever, malaise, and headache. The temperature usually ranges from 102° to 105° F, and malaise is severe. Frequently there is some mental confusion or clouding, which, like the headache, may be partly a general sign and partly a sign of involvement of the meninges and the underlying brain.

The specific **meningeal signs** are those due to irritation of the meninges. These vary from mild nuchal rigidity (splinting of the neck on forward flexion of the head) and the presence of Kernig's sign to the position of opisthotonus when these meningeal signs are developed to the fullest.

The **signs of cerebral involvement** include convulsions, mental confusion, and focal neurologic signs (the latter depend on the location of the meningeal exudate and the approximate amount and degree of involvement of the underlying brain tissue).

Specific signs referable to the type of meningitis are often present in meningococcal meningitis. There are petechiae in the skin (the rash of meningococcal meningitis). In addition, stroking the skin produces the tache cérébrale. In patients with other forms of meningitis, careful and complete examination reveals the focus of infection giving rise to the meningitis. The presence of an otitis media, signs of resolving pneumonia in the chest, or draining osteomyelitis all alert the examiner to the possible origin of the meningitis.

The most important **laboratory studies** in patients with meningitis are those derived from the cerebrospinal fluid. The lumbar puncture in patients with purulent meningitis reveals an increase in cerebrospinal fluid pressure ranging from 200 to 750 mm H_2O or more. The fluid varies from opalescent to purulent in color. The cell count reveals 500 to 20,000 or more white cells per cubic millimeter. Particularly in the earlier and acute stages of the disease, the cells are exclusively or chiefly polymorphonuclear in type. The total protein content is elevated and varies from 50 to 1,000 mg/100 ml. Protein content over 1,000 mg suggests that a block has developed in the cerebrospinal fluid system. The sugar in the spinal fluid is decreased and may not even be measurable. The abnormalities of colloidal gold are usually in the midzone and merely represent the increase of the total protein content.

Of greatest importance from the standpoint of treatment is the definition of the type of purulent meningitis present. This is contingent on the demonstration by smear and culture of the nature of the invading organism. Especially important are the studies of sensitivity of the offending organism to various antibiotics.

Other laboratory tests merely indicate the presence of an inflammatory disease. These include the elevated white blood cell count and the increased level of hematocrit. Blood cultures are helpful, particularly if the organisms are blood borne to the meninges.

Radiologic studies are not of value except in the elucidation of the presence of foci of infection elsewhere, such as in the nasal sinuses, mastoids, or lung fields.

The **treatment** of purulent meningitis must be early and vigorous. As soon as spinal fluid cultures have been inoculated, broad-spectrum antibiotics and sulfonamide drugs should be given, even though later the culture and sensitivity tests may change the choice of medication. The most widely used of the sulfonamide drugs is sulfadiazine. The antibiotics include penicillin, streptomycin, and chlortetracycline (Aureomysin). In all of these antimicrobial regimens, the aim is to maintain a sufficient concentration in the bloodstream to affect the organism. It is important to determine early the nature and sensitivity of the organism present and to administer the appropriate therapy.

In the therapy of meningococcal meningitis, sulfadiazine and penicillin are most widely used, sulfadiazine holding a particular advantage. Gonococcal meningitis is also best treated with sulfadiazine and penicillin. The meningitis caused by *Micrococcus catarrhalis* is best treated with sulfadiazine supplemented by an antibiotic, preferably oxytetracycline (Terramycin). Penicillin is the drug of choice in treating patients with pneumococcal meningitis. It is wise to augment this with sulfadiazine. Streptococcal meningitis is treated with antibiotics. Penicillin is most effective, and sulfadiazine is used as an added form of therapy. For patients with staphylococcal meningitis, penicillin, streptomycin, chlortetracycline, tetracycline, chloramphenicol, methicillin, and bacitracin may all be necessary, in that order of usage. Aureomycin and Terramycin are usually effective. In the treatment of patients with influenza meningitis, chloramphenicol may also be used if necessary, but with caution.

Although these are general outlines for the agents most likely to be effective in a case of purulent meningitis, for the particular patient it is necessary to determine the sensitivity for the invading organisms. Only in this way is it possible to determine the most advantageous drug for individual treatment. It is also important, whenever possible, to determine the blood levels of the therapeutic agent, to be certain that an adequate dosage is being used. Rapid advances in the treatment of infective diseases constantly alter the methods of management of the meningitides.

In the earlier days of antibiotic and chemotherapeutic attacks on the meningitides, it was customary to use intrathecal therapy. At present there seems to be little reason for this approach, since it is hazardous and may produce severe complications and since the establishment of an adequate blood level by parenteral or oral dosage usually suffices.

Meningitis in infants, especially influenza meningitis, may be complicated by subdural effusions, which can be diagnosed by subdural taps. If subdural effusions are persistent for an extended period, they should be treated by neurosurgical evacuation and removal of the membranes.

Nonpurulent leptomeningitis

The nonpurulent leptomeningitides are subacute or chronic. **Clinically** the patients present with a relatively low-grade fever, mild nuchal rigidity, malaise, and usually diffuse aching pain. Cranial nerve signs may be present. These patients, often without focal neurologic signs, are frequently seen in the medical wards as patients with unexplained fevers. Only the presence of meningeal signs suggests the need for a lumbar puncture. Since the meningeal signs may be slight, it is important to study the cerebrospinal fluid in all cases of unexplained fever. The presence of cells in the spinal fluid points the way to the proper diagnosis.

The nonpurulent leptomeningitides are essentially systemic. The differential diagnosis in this group includes treponemal (syphilis and leptospirosis); bacterial (tuberculosis); viral (benign lymphocytic choriomeningitis, Coxsackie, ECHO, and mumps); mycotic (torulosis and coccidiosis—rare); and meningeal involvement secondary to poliomyelitis, encephalitis, or brain abscess.

The latter three diagnoses are not primarily meningitides. The problem here is to determine whether the meningeal involvement is secondary to a parenchymal disease of the nervous system.

The diagnosis of **tuberculous meningitis** is based on the following features: a history of exposure to tuberculosis, evidence of tuberculosis elsewhere in the patient, and cerebrospinal fluid studies. In tuberculous meningitis there is a moderate increase in the spinal fluid pressure. The fluid is opalescent and may contain 25 to 500 cells, chiefly lymphocytes. The protein content is elevated from 45 to 500 mg/100 ml or more. There is also a progressive reduction in the sugar content. It is important to note that in the cell count there are usually 5% to 25% polymorphonuclear cells but rarely more than 50%. The final diagnosis depends on a demonstration of the tubercle bacillus in smear, culture, or guinea pig inoculation. Culture media for tubercle bacilli include Sabouraud's media, which also has the advantage of being a suitable culture growth for torulae.

The treatment of tuberculous meningitis is based on the use of streptomycin, isoniazid, and para-aminosalicylic acid. Streptomycin is suppressive but not eradicative; therefore isoniazid and para-aminosalicylic acid are also employed.

Syphilitic meningitis is discussed under neurosyphilis on pp. 153 and 154.

Torulosis of the leptomeninges is relatively uncommon. Torulosis may occur as a terminal feature in patients with debilitating diseases, especially in those with the lymphomas. The clinical features of torulosis of the meninges are the same as those in patients with other low-grade nonpurulent meningitides. In addtion to the preceding findings, examination of the spinal fluid shows organisms with the double refractile contour. These may be mistaken for red blood cells until the greater size of the torulae is recognized and the double refractile contour is noted. India ink study of the spinal fluid unequivocally demonstrates the torulae. Treatment consists of the use of amphotericin B.

Benign lymphocytic choriomeningitis

In patients with benign lymphocytic choriomeningitis there is often a history of exposure to rodents, particularly ones that died spontaneously. Sometimes the vector is not a rodent but an ordinary domestic animal. In this illness the prodromal symptoms develop five to ten days after exposure and have a duration of seven to twenty days. The symptoms are temperature that varies from 100° to 103° F and usually occurs in waves, malaise, general fatigue, generalized pain, and muscular weakness. An upper respiratory infection occasionally occurs from one to two weeks before the onset of meningitis. Early in the prodromal illness there is a definite leukopenia with granulopenia and a relative lymphocytosis. Involvement of the nervous system is manifested about twenty-three days after exposure to the virus and is characterized by an acute onset of fever, headache, and vomiting. The meningeal reaction lasts from seven to thirty days, gradually recedes, and is followed by recovery. Temperature varies from 101° to 104° F and is associated with chilliness. Usually the symptomatology is diffused and generalized, however. Meningeal signs are almost always present. Focal neurologic findings are rare but may be produced by parenchymal involvement, especially of the third and sixth cranial nerves.

The spinal fluid of patients with choriomeningitis is slightly turbid and under normal or slightly increased pressure. The cell count varies from 63 to 3,200 cells per cubic millimeter, and the cells are usually lymphocytes (95% to 100%). The spinal fluid sugar is generally normal, although there are patients in whom the sugar content is decreased to 35 mg/100 ml or less. This lowered sugar content may be persistent over a long period of time, as much as six to twelve months, after the acute illness is over. The protein content is elevated from 50 to 200 mg/100 ml. In all patients with nonpurulent meningitis, it is advisable immediately to draw 10 ml of sterile blood, which should be allowed to clot and be placed in the refrigerator. At a later date, if other causes have been ruled out, it is then possible to draw another 10 ml of blood and have the complement fixation titers determined on both the original blood serum and on this sample drawn two weeks later. If an increasing titer to the causative virus can be established a proper diagnosis is readily made.

No specific medications for patients with lymphocytic choriomeningitis are available at present, and therapy is therefore symptomatic. Few deaths are reported.

Enteroviral meningitides

The enteroviruses—ECHO, poliovirus, and Coxsackie—are common causes of meningitis. The poliovirus may produce only a meningitis (nonparalytic poliomyelitis) and therefore spare the neurons of the neuraxis. When this occurs **clinically,** the meningitis of poliovirus is indistinguishable from the ECHO, Coxsackie, and benign lymphocytic types. The occurrence of pleurodynia, herpangina, and pericarditis indicate a Coxsackie virus as the **etiologic agent.** Diarrhea may be a feature of ECHO virus infection. Respiratory infection and exanthemas occur in patients with both ECHO and Coxsackie infections.

The **diagnosis** of the enteroviruses is made on the basis of recovery of the particular virus from the stool or pharynx and serologic tests for neutralizing antibody.

Pachymeningitis

Pachymeningitis may be purulent or nonpurulent, cranial or spinal. Cranial purulent pachymeningitis occurs as either an epidural or subdural abscess and is the result of trauma or an osteomyelitis that is secondary to sinusitis or otitis media. These abscesses consist of a pocket of pus between the bone and the dura (epidural) or between the dura and the leptomeninges (subdural).

The **clinical signs** of pachymeningitis are fever, significant evidence of infection, a severe headache, which at first is localized, then generalized and followed by loss of consciousness, and focal neurologic signs depending on the site of the empyema. When purulent pachymeningitis occurs over the spinal cord, it is usually extradural and only rarely subdural. Here, too, it is generally secondary to osteomyelitis, with local back pain followed by root pain, due to compression of the nerve root, and if this is not heeded, by transverse myelitis due to the impairment of the blood supply to the spinal cord.

The **treatment** of the dural purulent meningitides is emergency surgical drainage followed by the proper chemotherapy for the particular organism.

The chronic types of pachymeningitis are tuberculous or syphilitic. Syphilitic pachymeningitis is extremely rare. The form most commonly described in neurologic literature occurs over the cervical cord (pachymeningitis cervicalis hypertrophica), resulting in the clinical picture of cord compression and therefore causing difficulty in differentiating it from a spinal cord tumor. Proper diagnosis is usually made on exploration.

Tuberculous pachymeningitis is generally spinal and associated with Pott's disease.

ENCEPHALITIS

Encephalitis is inflammation of the brain, and therefore, within its broader implications, brain abscesses are included. The inflammations of the brain other than brain abscess are divided according to etiology, that is, those due to viruses, rickettsiae, spirochetes, or other types of organisms.

Viral encephalitides

The viral encephalitides are a relatively newly understood group of diseases. Indeed, it was not until 1918 that they were recognized as such. The great pandemic of influenza that occurred during World War I with its concomitant encephalitis brought to physicians an awareness of this type of disease.

Encephalitis lethargica. Encephalitis lethargica was first described by von Economo. Although the **etiologic agent** has not been isolated, it is certain that the disease was of viral origin. Encephalitis lethargica occurred in epidemic form, probably beginning in isolated cases about 1915, assumed true epidemic proportions in 1917 and 1918, attained its peak in 1918 and 1919, and tapered off with the last definite cases occurring about 1925.

This disease affected people of all ages and of both sexes. The onset of malaise and fever was sudden, with or without a preceding respiratory infection of the influenza type. Disturbances of sleep patterns were common and characteristic of encephalitis lethargica. Most patients with this disease slept deeply and profoundly for days. However, the converse also occurred, and some patients were extremely restless and slept very little. Also, in some patients a day-night sleep reversal occurred. These alterations of sleep mechanism were probably produced by lesions of the reticular substance. Disturbances of ocular movements were common. Indeed, a permanent paralysis of convergence occurred in a great number of patients. The ocular palsies were often more obvious, and thus the onset of the illness could be with diplopia because of nuclear involvement of the oculomotor, trochlear, or abducens nuclei. In children convulsive seizures occurred early and often persisted as a sequela of the disease. Meningeal signs were prominent in some patients, and in fact, the clinical picture in many patients was predominantly meningitic.

The **pathologic lesions** in patients with encephalitis lethargica consisted of neuronal loss in the brain stem nuclei, lymphocytic meningitis, and evidence of inflammation of the brain with perivascular lymphocytic cuffing of the vessels in the white matter. Neuronal loss occurred particularly in the substantia nigra, globus pallidus, ocular motor nerve nuclei, reticular substance, and periaqueductal gray matter.

The mortality was high in the epidemic of von Economo's type of encephalitis lethargica. Many patients who did recover had permanent sequelae, for example, postencephalitic parkinsonism. Behavioral disorders were common as sequelae in children. Compulsive tics, oculogyric crises, and myoclonus, for example, of the palate, were also noted.

Narcolepsy, consisting of severe attacks of sleepiness, even in the most stimulating circumstances, occurred as a sequela of encephalitis. Cataplexy (loss of muscle control and power when in emotionally laden situations) occurred in some patients with narcolepsy. Although encephalitis is the most common cause of narcolepsy, the syndrome can also be caused by trauma and brain tumors.

The most important **laboratory studies** in encephalitis lethargica were those performed on spinal fluid. The pressure might be slightly increased. Also in the spinal fluid there was a moderate increase in cells, chiefly lumphocytes, and a slight elevation of protein levels.

Although this disease seems to have run its course in the great pandemic, occasionally sporadic cases clinically resemble encephalitis lethargica very closely. Since the diagnosis is based on clinical features alone, it is not possible to prove that these are the same entities that occurred in the era of World War I.

St. Louis type of encephalitis. St. Louis encephalitis is a particular disease that occurred in the early and late 1930s in St. Louis, Missouri. The **etiologic agent** has been identified as a definite filterable virus. The mode of transmission is by way of an arthropod.

Pathologically the lesions of St. Louis encephalitis are similar to those of encephalitis lethargica, but focal petechial hemorrhages also occur in this disease. The changes are most prevalent in the thalamus and brain stem and involve both gray and white matter.

Clinically the features are those of a febrile disease with lassitude, headache, and sore throat. There are meningeal signs, nuchal rigidity, and Kernig's sign. There may be severe disturbances of consciousness with prolonged coma. When these are absent, confusion, restlessness, and delirium may be present. The mortality is high (between 20% and 25%), but there is a low incidence of permanent sequelae.

Equine encephalomyelitis. Equine encephalomyelitis also is an arthropod-borne encephalitis. It occurs in two types due to two different viruses. These are known as the Western type, which has a lower mortality (20%), and the Eastern type, which is a more serious disease with a mortality of 74%. Of the patients with the Eastern type, virtually all survivors have serious sequelae. The latter disease cannot be differentiated clinically from the other encephalitides described herein.

Clinically there is evidence of a febrile disease, disturbance in consciousness, and other neurologic signs. A similar disease occurs in South America (Venezuelan equine encephalomyelitis) and is due to a virus separate and distinct from those causing the Eastern and Western types.

California virus encephalitis. California virus encephalitis is an arthropod-borne virus disease that is now recognized as occurring throughout much of the United States. It affects children, especially in rural areas. The clinical signs include fever, headache, lethargy, nausea, vomiting, stiff neck, occasionally convulsions, and rarely incoordination.

Japanese encephalitis. Japanese encephalitis occurs not only in Japan but also in China and Okinawa. This, also, is caused by an arthropod-borne virus.

Pathologically, Japanese encephalitis shows diffuse involvement of the brain. The disease occurs in late summer or early fall and has no distinguishing features in its clinical picture.

Russian tick-borne encephalitis. Russian Far East encephalitis is due to an arthropod-borne virus and occurs in spring and early summer. **Clinically** it is similar to the other encephalitides described, except that pronounced motor weakness occurs in these patients, particularly in the muscles of the neck and shoulder girdle.

Herpes simplex encephalitis. The virus of herpes simplex may cause an encephalitis that clinically may be similar to other types in onset. However, the virus has a special affinity for the temporal lobes and the limbic system, and therefore aphasia and other temporal lobe signs are common. This often leads to confusion in the diagnosis, and temporal lobe abscesses or tumors are considered likely. Seizures are often a prominent part of the **clinical condition.** Hemiparesis is also common. This disease may affect infants as well as adults and may occur in the first month of life, probably acquired from maternal genital herpes simplex lesions.

Examination of the spinal fluid reveals a lymphocytosis, usually between 50 and 200 cells per cubic millimeter. The protein content is moderately elevated and the sugar content may be decreased.

The outstanding **pathologic characteristic** is the presence of intraneuronal and intraglial inclusion bodies of the Dawson type A. However, these are not pathognomonic, since they occur in other virus diseases also.

The diagnosis can only be made with certainty by isolation of the virus from brain tissue. Serologic tests, demonstrating a progressive increase in antibody titer, are helpful but need to be interpreted with caution.

In herpes encephalitis the electroencephalogram presents a disorganized background with repetitive complexes occuring from 1 to 5 seconds and lasting 2 or 3 seconds, often most noticeable over the temporal lobe.

Herpes zoster. The virus that produces herpes zoster is similar to the virus of varicella. The disease occurs chieflly in adults.

The usual **clinical feature** of herpes zoster is the appearance of vesicular lesions of dermatomal distribution either on the trunk or the extremities or of trigeminal nerve distribution. These lesions are associated with severe pain and tenderness and occasionally even with motor weakness.

Pathologically the lesions are located in the dorsal root ganglion and the posterior roots of the spinal cord or the gasserian ganglion, but they may be more extensive and involve the motor roots also. Rarely, in addition to the skin lesions, the herpes zoster virus may cause a true encephalitis indistinguishable from the other encephalitides mentioned except, of course, for the occurrence of the herpetiform lesions.

Rabies. Rabies is an acute fatal encephalitis due to the bite of a rabid animal, usually domestic. However, various non-domestic mammals, including bats, may be rabid and transmit the disease by biting a human being. Rabies is an extremely severe encephalitis with widespread nerve cell loss and inflammatory changes involving the entire neuraxis. Characteristically there are inclusion bodies in the involved nerve cells (Negri bodies). The disease begins two to six weeks or longer after the inoculation of the virus. The duration of the incubation period depends on the amount of virus injected and the location of the skin lesion.

Clinically, in addition to the usual encephalitic picture, there are signs of extreme sensory irritation with painful spasms that occur when the patient attempts to swallow and with stimuli-induced convulsions.

Cytomegalic inclusion body encephalitis. Cytomegalic inclusion body encephalitis is an entity caused by a salivary gland virus. It occurs in patients in the neonatal and later periods. When this disease has its onset in the prenatal period, there is widespread systemic involvement with enlargement of the liver and spleen, jaundice, hemorrhages, convulsions, and prematurity. When it occurs in persons in later childhood (and rarely in those in adult life), this disease produces progressive evidence of brain damage with ataxia, myoclonic seizures, spasticity, and chorioretinitis. The diagnosis can be made by the demonstration of basophilic inclusion bodies in the epithelial cells present in urinary sediment and occasionally in gastric washings.

Rare forms of viral encephalitis. Psittacosis viral encephalitis is caused by a virus carried by infected parrots. **Cat-scratch fever** is an uncommon disorder. The virus of **lymphogranuloma venereum** may also cause encephalitis.

Slow viral infections

In the classic viral infections of the central nervous system (for example, in von Economo's encephalitis), the delay in onset between the acute illness and the occurrence of persistent neurologic sequelae (for example, parkinsonism), the steady progression of the course of the sequelae, and the demonstration at autopsy years later of perivascular infiltration all suggested a continuum of the infectious process. It is only in recent years, however, that the concept of slow viral infection has had its impact on neuropathologic and clinical neurologic thinking. The demonstration of transmissiblity of the etiologic agent in Jakob-Creutzfeldt disease has been noted on p. 105. There is a suggestion of transmissibility, perhaps by cannibalism, of kuru, a progressive ataxia with dyskinesia, dementia, paralysis, and incontinence occurring among the Fore people of the New Guinea highlands.

Subacute sclerosing panencephalitis is an uncommon, nonfamilial disease of the first two decades of life. Clinically it is characterized by dementia, seizures, especially myoclonic, dystonic movements, and increasing muscular rigidity. The electroencephalogram shows regularly spaced spiking dysrhythmias, which appear generalized but in time disappear. The course is progressive and fatal. The spinal fluid gamma globulin content is increased.

By electron microscopy viral particles were identified in the brains of children with this disease, and these viruses have been found to be similar to the measles virus. This finding correlates well with the rising titer of measles antibody in the serum of many of these patients. The observations indicate a pathologic slow viral activity of the measles virus on the central nervous sytem and open many opportunities for future investigations, not only in the infectious area of diseases of the central nervous system but also in diseases previously considered degenerative such as kuru and spastic pseudosclerosis (Jakob-Creutzfeldt). Hopefully, also, these and other studies will lead to a solution of the greatest enigma of modern neurology—multiple sclerosis.

Postinfectious or postexanthematous encephalomyelitides

The postinfectious or postexanthematous encephalomyelitides are also known as the perivenous demyelinating encephalomyelitides.

The **etiology** is probably based on an antigen-antibody relationship. The exanthematous diseases that may be followed by this encephalomyelitis are rubella, rubeola, varicella, and variola. Mumps also may be the cause. Vaccinations, particulary for variola and rabies and less commonly for pertussis, may also produce this type of encephalitis.

Pathologically these encephalomyelitides feature primarily the destruction of myelin in patches about blood vessels, especially veins. This occurs in the cerebrum, brain stem, and spinal cord.

Clinically the encephalomyelitis usually occurs about the tenth day after vaccination or in patients with exanthematous diseases as long as six days after the disappearance of the rash. The onset is usually abrupt with a recurrence of fever, disturbances of consciousness, convulsive seizures, muscular weakness, incoordination, and ataxia. The course of the disease is fairly rapid. Mortality figures vary and may be as high as 58%.

Acute disseminated encephalomyelitis

Acute disseminated encephalomyelitis is similar to the postinfectious encephalomyelitides, except that there is no antecedent history of vaccination or of an exanthematous disease.

Rickettsial encephalitides

Rickettsial encephalitides are uncommon. There are four main forms: Q fever, Rocky Mountain spotted fever, scrub typhus (tsutsugamushi disease), and typhus fever itself. Q fever presents evidence of a systemic disease and atypical pneumonia, occasionally with meningeal signs, numbness of the hands, nervousness, and insomnia. The latter suggest that there may be an encephalitis associated with Q fever. Rocky Mountain spotted fever is transmitted by tick bite. In the course of the systemic disease with exanthematous lesions, there may be severe central nervous system signs with disturbances of consciousness, meningeal signs, headaches, photophobia, and in children, convulsions. The rickettsial encephalitides are **treated** with the tetracycline antibiotics.

Spirochetal encephalitides

The various types of neurosyphilis, especially paresis, are discussed under neurosyphilis on pp. 151 to 154.

In **leptospirosis (Weil's disease)** the usual clinical picture includes meningeal signs, and evidence of cerebral involvement, such as restlessness, delirium, coma, and convulsions, may occur. Indeed, in rare cases these may occur without evidence of liver disease. Rat-bite fever and relapsing fever are rare causes of encephalitis.

Encephalitis due to protozoa

In the course of **malarial** infestations, especially those due to estivo-autumnal or malignant tertian malaria, the clinical picture of **cerebral malaria** may occur. Cerebral malaria is characterized by general premonitory signs, including those of febrile disease plus headache, vomiting, backache, nuchal pain, and vertigo and photophobia followed by localizing signs, such as hemiplegia, aphasia, or ataxia.

Toxoplasmosis is transmitted by domestic rodents. The mode of transmission is unknown. In adults there are usually no cerebral symptoms, and the disease manifests itself as a febrile illness with either or both pulmonary and cutaneous evidence. If, however, the adult is a pregnant woman, the disease may be transmitted by way of the placenta to the fetus. If this occurs early in gestation, the fetus may die, may have various anomalies such as hydrocephalus, microcephalus, or porencephaly, or may survive but be retarded and have convulsions. Chorioretinitis and cerebral calcification occur.

Toxoplasmosis may also occur in the adult in terminal stages of malignancies or when immunosuppressive therapy is used, for example, after organ transplantation.

Trypanosomiasis

Trypanosomiasis is a rare disease occurring in the inhabitants of South America (Chagas' disease) and also of Africa (sleeping sickness).

Helminthic encephalitis

Helminthic encephalitis is extremely rare in the United States. Trichinosis is probably the most common form but is rare.

BRAIN ABSCESS

Abscesses of the brain, either cerebral or cerebellar, are not primary but are always secondary to infection elsewhere. With the development of better treatment of those lesions that give rise to cerebral abscesses, the incidence of these intracranial infections has decreased rapidly.

The **etiology** of brain abscess is the implantation of organisms. The simplest mechanism for the development of brain abscess is direct implantation such as occurs in patients with penetrating head injuries. This is a rather infrequent cause, particularly in civil life. Brain abscesses may also occur from the direct extension of infection from contiguous structures, such as frontal sinuses and the mastoid air cells. In general, brain abscesses tend to arise from chronic, long-standing, severe sinusitis of the frontal sinuses and from relatively acute middle ear infections with mastoiditis. The spread of infection from the paranasal sinuses to the cerebral or cerebellar substance may be directly by osteomyelitis. The infection spreads across the dura and the subdural space directly to the brain. More commonly, however, the spread is by a process of thrombophlebitis or by metastases from distant lesions, for example, in the lung.

Pathologically a brain abscess consists of three parts—the innermost core and two layers of encapsulation. The core contains organisms and debris. The innermost layer of the capsule comprises new fibrous tissue, and distal to this is old fibrous tissue. Therefore the natural healing process is toward the center. The degree of encapsulation depends on the age of the abscess and the type of organism. Sometimes when the abscess is caused by highly virulent organisms, no capsule forms, and the abscess is a frank diffuse cerebritis. When an abscess approaches the ventricle, rupture may occur into the ventricle, since the ependymal cells have no restrictive ability.

If the abscess approaches the subarachnoid space, however, the leptomeninges, by employing their reparative functions, tend to seal it off.

The **clinical picture** of brain abscess consists of the signs of the primary disease, the general signs of brain abscess, and the local signs. When the primary disease is acute mastoiditis, the primary disease symptomatology is obvious. When nasal sinusitis is the cause, the signs and symptoms may be more obscure, since the sinusitis is generally chronic. Usually pulmonary infections are obvious when they give rise to brain abscess. Cardiac lesions, especially bacterial endocarditis, may be occult. The presence of cardiac murmurs (especially those suggesting congenital heart disease) and petechiae are suggestive of secondary brain abscess.

The general signs of brain abscess are those of infection and of intracranial hypertension, fever, apathy, and bradycardia. Intracranial hypertension occurs only when an abscess is extremely large or is so placed as to interfere with cerebrospinal fluid circulation. The febrile response in patients with brain abscess is usually moderate. The temperature may be no higher than 101° to 102° F. Apathy, indifference, and bradycardia are characteristic findings in the patient with brain abscess.

The local signs of brain abscess depend on its location. When the primary infection is in the mastoid cells, the abscess may occur either in the temporal lobe or in the cerebellum. Abscesses derived from frontal sinusitis are usually in the frontal lobe near the pole. Metastatic abscesses may occur anywhere but are most common in the distribution of the middle cerebral arteries, since this is the most direct route for infected emboli. Metastatic abscesses are usually multiple. Abscesses within the cerebellum produce ataxia and dyssynergia in the use of the extremities of the same side. They seldom cause cerebellar speech disturbances. The fourth ventricle may be compressed, therefore producing increased intracranial pressure early in its course; the medulla may also be compressed. Abscesses of the cerebrum produce hemiparesis, aphasia, and visual field defects, depending on their location. Seizures usually occur only in the early stages of brain abscess.

Of the **laboratory studies,** routine skull radiography is of little value in diagnosing brain abscess, except in demonstrating the primary inflammatory diseases of the nasal sinuses or the mastoid cells. The only other possible finding in the routine skull film is the shift of a calcified normal structure such as the pineal body.

The CT, or CAT, scan is of special value in the study of patients with a brain abscess, since pneumoencephalography carries with it some risk of inducing rupture of the abscess.

The cerebrospinal fluid examination of patients with brain abscess may show an increased pressure, indicating an expanding lesion and, in addition, show an aseptic meningeal reaction indicating an inflammatory process. There is a mild or moderate increase in cells with at least the presence of some polymorphonuclear cells. The total protein content in the fluid is also increased. The sugar content is normal.

Electroencephalographic studies may aid in localization, particularly if the abscess is near or in the cerebral cortex on the lateral surfaces of the hemispheres.

Treatment of patients with brain abscesses is both medical and surgical. Medical therapy is primarily directed at the control of the organism. In general, the same principles apply here as those discussed in the treatment of purulent meningitis. The choice of medication and dosage is the same. Since in many instances the exact organism is not known, broad-spectrum therapy is indicated. Surgical therapy should not be undertaken without adequate antimicrobial therapy. Generally one should not rush into surgical therapy. If the condition of the patient warrants, it is always better to treat the patient conservatively and thoroughly from the antibiotic and chemotherapeutic standpoint to permit the development of a capsule before surgical intervention is attempted.

POLIOMYELITIS

Poliomyelitis, or acute anterior poliomyelitis, has as its **etiology** a particular virus occurring in three serologic types. The mode of infection is usually by way of the nasopharynx, but it may also be by the gastroenteric route.

As the name implies, the chief **pathologic lesions** occur in the anterior gray matter of the spinal cord (ventral horns), where the motor nerve cells are present. There is partial loss of these neurons. Many of the remaining cells are in various stages of degeneration. Marked lymphocytic infiltration and proliferation of the microglia in the gray matter, perivascular lymphocytic cuffing in the white matter, and lymphocytic infiltration of the leptomeninges also occur. A characteristic of the lesions of the motor nerve cells is patchiness; that is, in sections of the cord the lesions may be profuse in one segment and minimal in the adjacent section, then again proceeding to various degrees of severity. This patchiness not only is present along the longitudinal axis of the cord but also in the cross section of the cord. With careful scrutiny of the anterior horns, one can often find a number of cells that are virtually normal in the midst of significant infiltration.

Although the term "acute anterior poliomyelitis" indicates the hallmark of the disease, the pathologic process is by no means limited to the anterior horns of the spinal cord. The posterior horns may also be involved. However, of much greater importance is the involvement of the bulbar motor nerve nuclei. The same lesions may also be present in the nuclei of the basal ganglia and the thalamus and occasionally even in the cerebral cortex. However, the greatest impact of this disease is on the ventral horns of the spinal cord and secondly on the bulbar motor nuclei.

Poliomyelitis occurs primarily in children and young adults. It is rare in infants in the first 6 months of life. Although the disease is uncommon in elderly and middle-aged persons, older people are certainly not excluded. The disease is more common in late spring, summer, and fall, although sporadic cases occur in the winter.

The usual **clinical picture** is that of an upper respiratory infection that subsides, followed in a period of one or two weeks by the onset of fever, malaise, mild stiffness of the neck, and headache. In patients with paralytic poliomyelitis, paralytic symptoms quickly follow. The paralysis is patchy and correlates well with the pathologic process. Massive paralysis of truncal and extremity muscles is rare. Usually segments of muscles are impaired; indeed, isolated muscle groups within a total muscle bulk are sometimes affected. There is muscle spasm of the affected muscles. No definite sensory changes are evident. The deep tendon reflexes are lost in the involved muscles and may be somewhat hyperactive elsewhere. Occasionally, positive plantar signs occur. Since the only possible reactive result to a noxious stimulus is dorsiflexion when the plantar flexors of the great toe are paralyzed, the positive plantar signs may be false. Abnormal plantar signs also may be produced by the transient edema of the white matter of the spinal cord. Urinary retention may occur in patients in the early phases of disease. If the bulbar nuclei are involved, paralysis or weakness or respiration, phonation, swallowing, and vocalization occur. This involvement is most critical, since life itself is threatened. With bulbar nuclei improvement, hypoxia may lead to mental confusion.

The most important **laboratory studies** are those of the spinal fluid. There is a moderate increase in cells. Within the first 24 hours after onset, the increase is predominantly polymorphonuclear but quickly becomes lymphocytic in type. The protein content is moderately elevated, and the sugar content is normal. Isolation of the virus from pharynx and stool and serologic identification help to document the etiology.

The most important **treatment** is preventive. Since the use of poliomyelitis vaccine has become widespread, this disease occurs infrequently. It is obvious that by judicious use of inoculation this disease can become as rare as smallpox.

There is no specific treatment. Once the disease is under way, it is impossible to change its course with specific therapy.

Symptomatic therapy consists of alleviation of muscle

spasms during the acute phase and the respiratory care of the patient. Moist hot packs are helpful in relieving the muscular contractions. In the respiratory care of patients with bulbar or upper cervical and thoracic cord involvement, judicious and early use of respirator and tracheotomy are important. The physician should not wait until cyanosis occurs. Pooling of secretion in the nasopharynx and a decrease in vital capacity (hoarseness of voice clinically often indicates impairment of vital capacity) are prompt indications for a tracheotomy, the use of the respirator, and oxygen therapy. As soon as the acute phase is past, active pursuit of rehabilitation and physical medicine procedures are indicated.

NEUROSYPHILIS

The improved preventive measures against syphilis and the great advancement in the treatment of primary and secondary syphilis have reduced to a minimum the new cases of neurosyphilis seen at the present time. Moreover, the improvements in the treatment of neurosyphilis have reduced this formerly prevalent neurologic disease to the status of a rare entity. However, with the increased incidence of primary syphilis, the later forms of syphilis with central nervous system involvement are beginning to appear, especially the vascular types. Moreover, the **clinical picture** may include only a part of the classic symptomatology.

In the **diagnosis** of neurosyphilis, various serologic tests of blood and spinal fluid are of great importance. *Treponema pallidum* evokes the production of lipid (nontreponemal) and of treponemal antibodies. The nontreponemal tests are less specific and sensitive than the treponemal tests, but since they are easier to run and less expensive, they are used as a general screening. Such tests include the original Wassermann, Kahn, and VDRL tests. The fluorescent detection of treponemal antibodies (FTA-ABS) is used to confirm the diagnosis and to rule out false positive or negative nontreponemal tests.

Paresis

The synonyms for paresis are generalized paresis and generalized paralysis of the insane. It is a syphilitic meningoencephalitis characterized **pathologically** by plasma cells and lymphocytic infiltration of the leptomeninges and cerebral cortex. The cellular infiltration combined with the proliferation of the neuroglial cells gives the false appearance of increased cellularity of the cerebral cortex. Actually, the neuronal elements of the cerebral cortex are greatly decreased in number, and those remaining are in various states of disintegration. In addition to involvement of the cerebral cortex, there are similar lesions in the cerebellum, thalamus, and hypothalamus. After treatment there is resolution of the inflammatory aspects and pronounced residual atrophy of the cortex.

The **clinical picture** of paresis is divisible into neurologic and psychiatric manifestations. The **neurologic symptoms** include headache and seizures that may be focal or generalized. Symptoms of aphasia may be obvious or elicited only on examination. The neurologic manifestations include tremulousness of the eyelids, lips, tongue, and fingers; slurred speech; hyperactive deep tendon reflexes; and positive plantar signs.

Psychiatric manifestations are chiefly those of organic mental deficit with impairment of memory (most prevalent for recent recall), lability of affect, impaired judgment, and impaired arithmetic ability. Although the expansive manic type of paresis is the classic psychiatric manifestation, this is not always present, and patients may show agitated depression and affective reaction. The coloring of the psychosis probably depends on the prepsychotic personality in this regard. Also, paresis may be of the simple, rapid, deteriorating type, probably related to a rapid, excessive encephalitic process.

The **cerebrospinal fluid** in patients with untreated paresis shows a normal or slightly increased spinal fluid pressure. The fluid is usually clear, and there is an increase in cells. Total protein content is moderately elevated; sugar content is normal. Colloidal gold reactions show a first zone abnormality. The gamma globulin content is also increased. The cerebrospinal fluid serology is positive. Blood serology is almost always positive.

Generalized paresis is an unremitting and fatal disease unless it is **treated.** Penicillin in massive doses administered intramuscularly (total of 25 million units) may be given at the rate of 1 to 1.5 million units/24 hr. In patients who are sensitive to penicillin, chlortetracycline can be used. The various types of fever therapy are no longer employed.

Tabes dorsalis

Pathologically tabes dorsalis is characterized by demyelination of the posterior columns of the spinal cord and the posterior roots, with the primary lesions probably in the dorsal root ganglia.

The **clinical picture** of tabes includes pain, which is characteristically lightninglike, occurs in bouts, and affects the extremities or the trunk. There is considerable loss of position sense, which gives rise to ataxia and ataxic gait. Because of the dorsal root involvement, the deep tendon reflexes are lost at the ankle and usually at the patella. There is also a decrease in muscle tone. Deep pain sensation is impaired so that the tendon of Achilles or the testicles can be squeezed without eliciting pain. The combination of hypotonia and loss of deep pain sensation probably is the chief factor causing the disintegration of joints (Charcot's joints), which commonly occurs in the extremities of patients with this disease. There are also peculiar bands of hypesthesias occurring in cuirass fashion over the thorax, sometimes in a butterfly distribution about the nose, and on the lateral aspects of arm, hand, leg, and foot (Hitzig's zones).

The **cerebrospinal fluid** pressure is normal. The fluid may contain a mild increase in cells, a slight increase in protein, some alteration of gold sol reaction, elevated gamma globulin, and positive serology. Tabes, however, unlike paresis, is a self-limiting disease. Even without treatment the spinal fluid may become normal ("burnt-out tabes").

Treatment of tabes follows the same pattern as that of paresis. There is some question as to the advisability of treating patients with burnt-out tabes. However, if they have not been given an adequate course of penicillin, it is usually customary to do so. Treatment of the lightninglike pains is frequently exceedingly difficult. Therapy may lead to narcotic addiction. Therefore the use of drugs such as nialamide is indicated. If the salicylates and the newer drugs fail to alleviate the pain, a cordotomy may be indicated.

Taboparesis

Many patients with either tabes or paresis show some combination of the two. These are merely admixtures of the two disease entities previously described.

Vascular neurosyphilis

Fortunately, vascular neurosyphilis also has become extremely infrequent. Syphilis **pathologically** causes an intimal proliferation in certain of the larger and medium-sized vessels of the brain. This progresses to an actual obliteration of these vessels, with infarction of the brain distal to the occluded vessel. This proliferation is most common in patients in the age group below 45 years. The **clinical picture** is that of encephalomalacia (Chapter 4). The **diagnosis** is made on studying the spinal fluid of the patient in the younger age group with a cerebrovascular accident. Findings on **spinal fluid** examination include increased white cell count, perhaps slight elevation of protein, positive serology, and increased gamma globulin content. **Treatment** is the same as that for general paresis.

Syphilitic meningitis

Syphilitic meningitis, formerly a relatively uncommon disorder, is now extremely rare. There are three types of syphilitic meningitis: (1) that occurring over the vertex of the brain, (2) that at the base of the brain, and (3) syphilitic hydrocephalus. In patients with syphilitic meningitis over the vertex, the presenting features are focal cerebral signs, for example, focal convulsions, hemiplegia, monoplegia, and language disturbance. Syphilitic meningitis at the base affects the cranial nerves, particularly the eighth, third, and sixth nerves. Acute syphilitic hydrocephalus is due to meningeal exudate blocking the lateral recess and the foramina of the point at the exit of the fourth ventricle. This causes an obstruction of the cerebrospinal fluid pathways with dilatation of the fourth ventricle, aqueduct, and lateral ventricles. The diagnosis is derived from the spinal fluid findings. The treatment is the same as that for paresis, except that neurosurgical procedures may be necessary to relieve the block.

REFERENCES

Alpers, B. J.: Treatment of neurosyphilis. In Forster, F. M., editor: Modern therapy in neurology, St. Louis, 1957, The C. V. Mosby Co.

Baker, A. B.: Viral encephalitis. In Baker, A. B., editor: Clinical neurology, ed. 3, New York, 1972, Harper & Row, Publishers, Inc.

Baker, A. B., and Cornwell, S.: Poliomyelitis. XV. The spinal cord, Arch. Pathol. **61:**185, 1956.

Bennett, D. R., Zu Rhein, G. M., and Roberts, T. S.: Acute necrotizing encephalitis: a diagnostic problem in temporal lobe disease, Arch. Neurol. **6:**96, 1962.

Fetter, F. B., et al.: Mycoses of the central nervous system, Baltimore, 1967, The Williams & Wilkins Co.

Finley, K. H.: The treatment of the encephalomyelitides. In Forster, F. M., editor: Modern therapy in neurology, St. Louis, 1956, The C. V. Mosby Co.

Hooshmand, H., et al.: Neurosyphilis: a study of 241 patients, J.A.M.A. **219:**726, 1972.

Meningitis, Int. J. Neurol. **4:** 1964.

Merritt, H. H., Adams, R. D., and Solomon, H. C.: Neurosyphilis, New York, 1946, Oxford University Press.

Ohya, T., et al.: SSPE—correlation of clinical, neurophysiologic and neuropathologic findings, Neurology (Minneap.) **24:**211, 1974.

Proceedings of First International Poliomyelitis Conference, Philadelphia, 1949, J. B. Lippincott Co.

Sahs, A. L.: Meningitis. In Baker, A. B., editor: Clinical neurology, ed. 3, New York, 1972, Harper & Row, Publishers, Inc.

Salk, J. E.: Poliomyelitis vaccination in the fall of 1956, Am. J. Public Health **47:**1, 1957.

Symposium on herpes simplex encephalitis, Postgrad. Med. J. **49:**1, 1973.

Symposium: Measles virus and subacute sclerosing panencephalitis, Neurology (Minneap.) **18:**1, 1968.

Thompson, W. H., and Evans, A. S.: California encephalitis virus studies in Wisconsin, Am. J. Epidemiol. **81:**230, 1965.

Zu Rhein, G. M., and Chou, S. M.: Particles resembling papova viruses in human cerebral demyelinating disease, Science **148:**1477, 1965.

11   Trauma to the nervous system

In view of the continuing urbanization and mechanization of American society and the continuing military threats, trauma to the nervous system assumes ever-increasing significance.

CRANIAL TRAUMA
Skull fracture

A fracture of the skull may be **simple,** that is, merely evidenced by radiographic examination and accompanied by few or no symptoms. A simple fracture in itself is not important except as an indication of the severity of the head injury. However, a simple skull fracture may assume grave importance from the standpoint of location. A fracture into the base of the skull may produce rhinorrhea or otorrhea, with the drainage of spinal fluid from the nose or ear and with possible development of meningitis as a sequel. A fracture through one of the paranasal sinuses carries the same threat of meningitis. A fracture across a major vessel groove such as that of the middle meningeal artery can cause an epidural hematoma. If fracture of the calvarium is associated with a laceration of the scalp **(compound fracture),** an easy entrance of organisms is permitted, and osteomyelitis, epidural abscess, or meningitis may follow. Either simple or compound fractures may be **depressed.** Because of the distortion of soft tissues by edema and hemorrhage, palpation alone is not sufficient to diagnose depression of fragments. Carefully produced radiographic films are essential.

Simple skull fracture requires no specific **therapy,** although it is customary, since it does indicate a severe head injury, to enforce a period of rest and decreased activity on the patient. This also makes it possible to observe the patient for evidence of developing neurologic signs. Patients with otorrhea or rhinorrhea should be kept propped up in bed in an attempt to decrease the intraventricular pressure as much as possible. To prevent the introduction of pathogenic organisms into the subarachnoid spaces, patients should be cautioned to avoid sneezing by pressing on the upper lip and should not be allowed to blow their noses. Careful observation should be made of their temperature and pulse rate. Prophylactic broad-spectrum antibiotics should be administered to avoid the possibility of meningitis. When rhinorrhea is persistent, it may be due to trapping of the meninges in the fractures through the cribriform plate. It may be necessary to have the dural defect in this area closed by intracranial neurosurgical procedure. Depressed fractures should be elevated as soon as possible.

Intracranial hematomas

Posttraumatic intracranial hematomas may develop either on the outer surface of the dura, dissecting the dura from the bone (**epidural** or **extradural hematoma),** or between the dura and the subarachnoid membrane (**subdural hematoma),** or within the substance of the brain (**intracerebral hematoma).** In patients with extremely severe head injuries, there may be massive, rapid bleeding into any or all of these sites.

Clinically there is usually an obviously severe head injury, generally associated with loss of consciousness and followed by a period of relative or complete freedom from neurologic signs and symptoms. Gradually neurologic symptoms reappear, including disturbance of consciousness, focal neurologic signs such as seizures, aphasia, and hemiplegia, or evidences of increased intracranial pressure. The evidence of increased intracranial pressure includes pupillary disturbances and headache. The signs and symptoms are characteristically somewhat remitting and exacerbating, depending on adjustment to the increased intracranial pressure and to the torsion exerted on the cerebral structures.

It is often difficult clinically to distinguish between the three types of hematomas. Subdural hematoma is most common, and intracerebral hematoma is least common. Epidural hematomas generally occur shortly after the injury, in a matter of hours to several days, since the bleeding is usually arterial. Occasionally as much as two weeks are required for the development, but then the resulting epidural hematoma is usually venous in origin.

Laboratory studies in patients with hematomas or suspected hematomas include electroencephalography, radiographic examinations including contrast studies, CAT scans, and isotopic studies. The electroencephalogram may show significant slowing in the area of the hematoma but may also be deceptively normal, the hematoma contents being able to transmit the normal electroencephalogram and the hematoma not being sufficiently large to have embarrassed the brain function. In epidural hematomas, x-ray films of the skull will demonstrate a fracture line crossing the middle meningeal groove. The absence of pineal shift is not a reliable indicator for the absence of a hematoma. Likewise, on angiography, midline position of the anterior cerebral arteries does not rule out the presence of subdural hematomas. Since subdural hematomas are often bilateral, midline structures may not be shifted. The important laboratory test is the demonstration of a space between the peripheral cortical small vessels and the inner surface of the cranium.

The **treatment** for all posttraumatic intracranial hematomas is the neurosurgical evacuation of the hematoma as soon as a diagnosis is made and the patient's condition warrants, that is, when the patient is not in extreme surgical shock from the immediate head injury. The degree of trauma necessary to produce a subdural hematoma is sometimes almost negligible. For this reason the differentiation between cerebrovascular accident and subdural hematoma is sometimes impossible. When the diagnosis cannot be established, it is justifiable to recommend appropriate studies, especially angiography or exploration for a hematoma.

Lacerated and/or contused brain

Usually laceration or contusion of the cerebral cortex is accompanied by fracture and may coexist with a hematoma. These patients are often restless and manifest meningeal signs and focal neurologic signs. The cerebrospinal fluid is bloody or pink tinged. On microscopic examination the red blood cells are found to be crenated, indicating that they have been present for some time in the spinal fluid. The treatment of these patients is symptomatic, aimed at reducing the restlessness and increased intracranial pressure that often accompany laceration and contusion. Fluid restrictions are expedient. Careful attention should be given to electrolyte balance. Mild sedation or, preferably, tranquilizing agents of the meprobamate series are effective against restlessness.

Concussion

The definition of concussion is a syndrome produced by head injury, severe enough to cause a transient loss of consciousness without indication of any of the neurologic complications of head injury described in the preceding. It is not uncommon for patients with concussions to have a retrograde amnesia, a portion of which may be permanent.

Posttraumatic sequelae

Posttraumatic sequelae include epilepsy and the posttraumatic syndrome. Trauma is a most important cause of epileptic seizures. (See Chapter 6.)

The posttraumatic syndrome as a sequel of head injuries is more common after a closed head injury or the concussive type of head injury than after an open head injury. The syndrome consists of headaches, vertigo, memory defects, affect changes chiefly in the nature of irritability, easy fatigability, and occasionally vasomotor disturbances. These are usually present after the patient returns to consciousness. The symptoms tend to become progressively less evident and generally remit within six to twelve months, although parts or all of the syndrome may become permanent.

SPINAL CORD AND SPINAL ROOT TRAUMA

The three most important categories of spinal cord and spinal root trauma are fractures and fracture dislocations of the spine, ruptured intervertebral disks, and hematomyelia.

Fracture and fracture dislocations

Fracture and fracture dislocations are most common in the region of the cervical and lumbar spine and less common in the thoracic region because of the rigidity and protection of the thoracic cage, since the combination of vertebra, sternum, and ribs tends to make a composite whole. Fracture and fracture dislocations of the thoracic spine are possible, however. Most frequent of these are the compression fractures that occur in the course of convulsive seizures, particularly in patients receiving electroshock therapy. Vertebral fractures may also be spontaneous and due to metastatic carcinoma or multiple myelomas. A prime mechanism in producing cervical spine fractures and fracture dislocations is acute impact on the vertex of the head with the neck flexed and, especially, somewhat rotated. This is the usual mechanism of football cervical cord injuries, as well as many cord injuries occurring in automobile accidents.

Although severe trauma to the spine may produce fracture or fracture dislocation, it is important to note that the dislocation may be rapidly self-reducing, so that at the time of radiographic examination the actual dislocation may no longer be evident.

The **clinical signs** are those of complete or partial transection of the spinal cord with interruption of all ascending modalities below the level of the lesion and of descending functions below that level. There may be, and frequently is, pain over the vertebra at the site of the injury. There may be, and frequently is, pain over the vertebra at the site of the injury. There may be root pains also at this level.

In the management of these patients it is necessary to determine whether a subarachnoid block exists. If so, spinal cord decompression is essential and is performed with the hope that a fragment of bone is compressing the cord or edema of the cord is giving rise to the block and the spinal cord symptoms. More often, however, the symptomatology is due to the injury wreaked on the cord at the time of trauma, often by the fracture dislocation. The cord itself is reduced to a softened myelomalacic mass. The surgical exploration is indicated, however, to reduce the amount of damage at this point due to swelling of the cord and further impairment of the blood supply by edema of the cord within the rigid spinal canal.

It is generally recognized that the treatment of the acute spinal cord injury must be immediate and well within a 4-hour period. If surgical decompression will accomplish anything, it will be within that time span, except for the rare instances of subdural spinal hematomas. Even in these, however, urgency is indicated. Various investigations are under way employing spinal cord cooling and the use of various enzymes to prevent the central gray matter necrosis that results from these injuries.

It is extremely important in handling these patients in the course of procedures, including radiographic examinations, to exercise the utmost care in moving the spine to avoid further severing or damaging the already traumatized spinal cord. When it is clear that no block is present, treatment is conservative, and various devices for immobilizing the spine are indicated. When feasible, as for patients with cervical fractures, traction is employed.

Herniated disk syndrome

Herniations of the intervertebral disk occur in the cervical and lumbar regions. Protrusions of the thoracic disks are uncommon but may occur after electroshock therapy or other thoracic spine trauma. They are most common in the lumbar region. Usually the history is of trauma, with acute onset of low back pain followed later by root pain in sciatic distribution.

The typical **clinical picture** includes decreased or absent deep tendon reflexes at the ankle or knee, depending on the level of the lesion, and a dermatome type of sensory loss, combined with splinting of the spine and a positive Lasègue sign (impaired straight leg raising). If the disk has been ruptured for a considerable length of time, a slight to moderate degree of atrophy may be present in the affected musculature, and fasciculations can be seen.

Herniated intervertebral disks of the cervical spine are somewhat less common than those in the lumbar region. The history of trauma is often not so clearly evident, and the diagnosis is more often confused with spinal cord tumor or the complications of osteoarthritis of the spine. Pain, when present, is in a cervical dermatome. There are long tract signs involving both upper and lower extremities, some decrease of mobility in the cervical spine, and reflex changes, and atrophy occurs in the region of cervical supply.

A diagnosis of ruptured intervertebral disk is dependent not only on the clinical signs and symptoms but also on radiographic and cerebrospinal fluid evidence. In disks that have been ruptured for some time, narrowing of the intervertebral spaces at the point of extrusion of the disk and loss of the usual cervical or lumbar curves in the lateral views radiographically are evident. The cerebrospinal fluid protein content is elevated and somewhat higher in patients with ruptured lumbar disks. A complete or partial block is extremely rare. Myelographic examination is helpful in the presence of a well-developed ruptured intervertebral disk syndrome and shows characteristic distortion of the column of radiopaque substance.

The **treatment** of herniated cervical intervertebral disks is difficult if the disk has been extruded for any length of time, since then the disk may be calcified and bony hard. Removal would be dangerous because of the possibility of traumatizing the cord. Neurosurgical procedures employed in such patients are laminectomy for increasing the size of the canal and section of the dentate ligaments to allow more freedom of motion of the spinal cord.

In the surgical treatment of ruptured cervical disk, many neurosurgeons prefer the anterior approach with the fusion of the two vertebrae, thus increasing the stabilization of the cervical spine, in contradistinction to laminectomy, which decreases the stability of the spine. Conservative methods such as traction may also be helpful. Herniated lumbar disk, when well defined, should be removed surgically, particularly in patients with occupations making recurrences likely and in instances in which the disk is giving sufficient incapacity. The first attack in a patient with a sedentary occupation can be treated with bed rest, salicylates, muscle relaxants, and heat therapy.

Diskolysis consists of the enzymatic dissolution of a ruptured intervertebral disk. This has been employed in the treatment of lumbar disk problems. However, the future of this approach is unclear, since the enzymatic dissolution may lead to arachnoiditis and bony destruction.

Hematomyelia

Hematomyelia is an uncommon but serious type of cord injury, **pathologically** consisting of multiple small perivascular hemorrhages in the spinal cord. Since the gray matter is more abundantly supplied with blood vessels, hemorrhages are more frequent in the gray than in the white matter.

The **clinical picture** is often delayed in onset. The injury is frequently a compressive type, followed after a period of several hours or a day by the onset of symptoms. The signs are those of partial to complete transverse section of the spinal cord, more frequently partial and more often with a preponderance of anterior horn cell signs, causing weakness, particularly in the upper extremities. Since the level of the hematomyeliac lesions in the spinal cord bears no relation to the actual site of the injury, a compression injury in the lumbar or thoracic area may give rise to cervical signs. Hematomyelia has no specific treatment.

General management of spinal cord injuries

There is probably nothing more taxing in the care of patients with neurologic diseases than the rehabilitative, nutritional, urinary, and skin management of the patient with transverse myelitis. The utmost care must be exercised to prevent acute decubiti. The maintanance of a dry, clean bed is paramount. Stryker frames, which permit frequent turning of the patient and prevent pressure for an undue time on one part, are a signal advance in therapy. Various types of continuous bladder drainage are helpful. Those types dependent on an indwelling catheter and tidal drainage have the added advantage of making possible the development of an automatic control of the bladder in some patients. When this is not feasible, a suprapubic cystostomy with an indwelling catheter is helpful. The rehabilitative factors require considerable skill on the part of the physician in maintaining motivation for the patient and guiding his intellectual assets into the most useful channel available to him.

TRAUMA TO PERIPHERAL NERVES

The peripheral nerves in the upper extremities are more frequently involved by trauma than are those of the lower extremities. The **brachial plexus** may be traumatized at birth if there is too forcible a deviation of the head on or away from the shoulder. Forcible deviation of the head at any time in life can traumatize the plexus. Either the upper or lower roots of the brachial plexus may thus be avulsed. If the upper segments are involved, the intrinsic muscles of the hand are still functioning well, but the shoulder muscles are weak. To flex their elbows, these patients "climb" their vest buttons with their fingertips. In contrast, when the involvement is primarily of the lower portion of the brachial plexus, the more distal muscles and the intrinsic muscles of the hand are affected. Brachial plexus injury at birth is associated with atrophy and wasting of the involved part.

The **long thoracic nerve** that supplies the serratus magnus muscle may be injured by carrying heavy objects on the shoulder. It may also be traumatized in contact sports, for example, by the charge of a lineman on the football team. The result of this injury is winging of the scapula when the arms are extended and adducted. This nerve subserves no cutaneous sensation. If there is pain in the shoulder with serratus magnus weakness, it is because of the weight of the winged scapula.

The **ulnar, radial,** and **median nerves** are commonly involved in trauma to the arm, forearm, and wrist area. The radial nerve is the extensor nerve in the upper extremity and by its innervation the fingers, wrist, and elbow are extended. Sensory innervation is most definite on the hand between the thumb and index finger. The radial nerve may be readily traumatized in its groove around the humerus (Saturday night paralysis).

The ulnar nerve may be affected immediately by injuries, or many years after an intercondylar fracture of the humerus, the groove for the ulnar nerve may be encroached on by abnormal callus formation. The most obvious functions of this nerve are the adduction and abduction of the fingers, apposition of thumb and little finger, and the ability to grasp flat objects (as a card) between the forefinger and the thumb. When this test is performed by a patient with ulnar nerve involvement, the interphalangeal joint of the thumb flexes and the thumb rotates against the index finger to grasp the card (Froment's sign). The best defined sensory innervation from the ulnar nerve is the skin of the little finger and at least the lateral half of the ring finger, projected from this point over both volar and palmar surfaces to the wrist. If the sensory loss extends beyond the wrist and up the arm, the lesion is more likely of the seventh and eighth cervical roots than of the ulnar nerve itself.

The median nerve is most often injuried in lesions at the wrist, particularly severing lesions occurring on the palmar aspect of the wrist or in the carpal tunnel syndrome. This nerve supplies the flexor muscles of the fingers. A simple, quick test for median nerve function is a rapid apposition of the thumb to the tips of each of the other fingers. The sensory supply is most definite over the distal two joints of the index and third and middle fingers on both volar and palmar surfaces.

A **quick survey** of the **status** of **these three main nerves** of the upper extremities may be made at the time of an injury or certainly before a cast is placed on the patient. Motor functions can be tested by flexion and extension of the fingers, abduction and adduction of the fingers. Sensory status can be evaluated by crisscrossing the hand on both volar and palmar surfaces with a pin, beginning on the base of the little finger and crossing to the base of the proximal interphalangeal joint of the thumb and from the base of the index finger to the base of the hypothenar eminence.

Trauma to the entire **sciatic nerve** is uncommon. It may occur, however, as the result of improperly administered intramuscular injections in the buttocks. The lesion of the entire sciatic nerve results in a paralysis of the whole lower extremity except for the functions of adduction of the thigh (obturator nerve), extension of the knee (femoral nerve), and extension of the thigh by the gluteal groups.

The **lateral peroneal nerve,** a branch of the sciatic, is the one in the lower extremity most commonly injured, since it may be traumatized by pressure on the lateral surface of the tibia. A cast to the lower leg can injure this nerve. Since it supplies the extensor muscles of the leg, lesions of it cause impairment of extension of the toes, dorsiflexion, and eversion of the foot, that is, foot drop.

The **tibial nerve,** which is the main flexor nerve of the leg and foot, is infrequently involved in trauma. When it is, impaired plantar flexion of the foot with atrophy of the anteromedial aspect of the calf occurs.

The **femoral nerve** supplying the quadriceps group of muscles is uncommonly affected. In lesions of this nerve, paralysis of extension of the knee occurs, making the patient unable to walk or stand.

REFERENCES

Brock, S.: Injuries of the skull, brain and spinal cord, ed. 2, Baltimore, 1943, The Williams & Wilkins Co.

Committee on Rating of Mental and Physical Impairment, Guides to evaluation of permanent impairment of peripheral spinal nerves, J.A.M.A. July, 1964.

Gurdjian, E. S., and Webster, J. E.: Head injuries: mechanisms, diagnosis, and management, Boston, 1958, Little, Brown & Co.

Pool, J. L.: The neurosurgical treatment of traumatic paraplegia, Springfield, Ill., 1951, Charles C Thomas, Publisher.

Prather, G. C., and Mayfield, F. H.: Injuries of the spinal cord, Springfield, Ill., 1953, Charles C Thomas, Publisher.

Trauma of the central nervous system, Proceedings of the Association held in New York, Assoc. Res. Nerv. & Ment. Dis., Proc. **24:**679, 1945.

Woodhall, B., and Beebe, G. W.: Peripheral nerve injuries, Veterans Administration Medical Monograph, 1956, Veterans Administration.

12 Diseases affecting the cranial and peripheral nerves

DISEASES AFFECTING THE CRANIAL NERVES
First cranial (olfactory) nerve

The first cranial (olfactory) nerve may be destroyed by a fracture of the cribriform plate, resulting in permanent anosmia. If the fracture is accompanied by rhinorrhea (dripping of spinal fluid from the nose), an urgent need for antibiotic therapy to prevent meningitis is indicated, and the patient should avoid sneezing, which might cause an inhalation of organisms with dissemination and infection of the leptomeninges. The olfactory nerve may be affected by brain tumors, particularly meningiomas arising from the cribiform plate. Sinusitis, however, can also cause anosmia.

Second cranial (optic) nerve

Neuritis and retrobulbar neuritis of the optic nerve are manifested by relatively acute loss of vision, which may be complete or partial. The decreased visual acuity, which may be unilateral or bilateral, is frequently described as "a cloud that came in front of the eye." Patients sometimes are subjectively aware of scotomas, which may be unilateral or bilateral. On funduscopic examination in patients with retrobulbar neuritis, no abnormalities are noted because the location of the lesion in the optic nerve is at some distance behind the optic disk. However, in a patient with optic neuritis, in whom the lesion is at or near the nerve head, the disk is elevated, with loss of the physiologic cup and congestion of veins, and there may be exudates but rarely hemorrhages. On appearance alone it is difficult, if not impossible, to distinguish between optic neuritis and papilledema due to increased intracranial pressure. If, however, the elevation is 5 diopters or greater, it is more likely to be due to papilledema than to optic neuritis. Also, extensive hemorrhages seldom occur in patients with optic neuritis.

The visual field examinations are exceedingly important in the differential diagnosis. In patients with papilledema the visual fields are slightly constricted peripherally, and the blind spot is enlarged because of the enlargement of the disk head by edema. By contrast, the field defect in patients with optic neuritis and retrobulbar neuritis consists of scotomas, usually paracentral; the scotoma may also affect the macular vision. When the eyes are moved, pain is present in patients with optic neuritis, especially in those with retrobulbar neuritis, but not in those with papilledema.

Abnormalities of the visually evoked potentials (VECA or VER) persist and are evidence of a preexisting optic neuritis or retrobulbar neuritis, even when the visual fields have returned to normal.

In patients with **optic atrophy,** the disk is pale, white or grayish, and sharply outlined. Primary optic atrophy may be caused by trauma when the optic nerve is severed by fracture at the foramen, or it may occur secondary to meningitis, particularly in patients with syphilitic meningitis. Formerly it was often seen in patients with tabes. Optic atrophy may occur secondarily to papilledema. It can also be caused by certain toxic agents, notably methyl alcohol or certain arsenical derivatives.

Third cranial (oculomotor), fourth cranial (trochlear), and sixth cranial (abducens) nerves

The third, fourth, and sixth cranial nerves may be involved in trauma, the third and sixth more commonly than the fourth. Osteomyelitis of the tip of the petrous temporal bone is no longer common, since mastoiditis is so rare, but in this process the sixth cranial nerve was often involved. However, in older patients with diabetes, isolated sixth nerve palsies occasionally occur and may be transient. These cranial nerves may be involved in the various meningitides. Also, these cranial nerves combined with the first sensory branch of the fifth cranial nerve may be involved in diseases affecting the cavernous sinus, such as the now rare cavernous sinus thrombosis and the uncommon carotid artery–cavernous sinus arteriovenous fistula. The latter is usually produced by trauma but may occur because of spontaneous rupture within the cavernous sinus of an aneurysm of the internal carotid artery.

Extraocular palsies may result from the rare, congenital neuronal defects of the nucleus of the sixth nerve (Möbius syndrome) or the fibrotic degeneration of the lateral rectus muscle (Duane syndrome).

Fifth cranial (trigeminal) nerve

The most common disease of the fifth cranial nerve is **tic douloureux.** This disease occurs in elderly persons, usually in the sixth decade or older. It is characterized by showers of sharp, stabbing, knifelike pains occurring in the distribution of the fifth cranial nerve. The pain may be in one or more branches of the nerve and may occur in paroxysms lasting several minutes and are often repeated frequently during the day. Tic douloureux may occur as a disease entity or secondary to herpes zoster infections in the fifth nerve distribution. It may be mimicked by dental problems. When a younger person appears to have tic douloureux, one must be especially careful to search for dental or other causes. Occasionally the syndrome of tic douloureux may be caused by neoplasms occurring near the sensory ganglion of the trigeminal nerve or within the paranasal sinuses.

The most effective drug in the treatment of tic douloureux is carbamazepine (Tegretol) and is administered in doses of 200 mg/three or four times a day. However, Tegretol may cause hematopoietic depression, and therefore regular blood studies should follow its use. Tegretol therapy should be reserved for definite cases of trigeminal neuralgia and preferably when other treatments fail. Other medical therapy in tic douloureux consists of inhalation of trichloroethylene drops placed on a handkerchief. This may tend to alleviate an attack. Sodium diphenylhydantoinate may be taken in doses of 0.3 Gm/24 hr or more as a preventive. In some patients nialamide (Niamid) may prevent attacks.

Many patients with tic douloureux, however, find surgical treatment necessary. The nerve may be blocked with alcohol. If this is unsuccessful or is successful for only a short time, resection of the appropriate sensory root is indicated.

Neuromas of the fifth cranial nerve are rare. Patients with neuromas present with trifacial pain, show other cranial nerve signs, and usually have an elevated spinal fluid total protein content.

Seventh cranial (facial) nerve

Bell's palsy is the most common involvement of the seventh cranial nerve. This is an acute paralysis of one side of the face. It occurs in persons in all groups but most frequently in adults. Bell's palsy may follow an infection or prolonged exposure to cold, but usually it is not associated with any obvious precipitating factor. The palsy may be moderate, may affect only part of the facial musculature, may vary somewhat in severity from branch to branch of the facial nerve, and may progress into complete paralysis of one side of the face. In patients with severe cases there is often hyperacusis of the ear on the affected side due to involvement of the nerve to the stapedius muscle. Taste may be lost on the same side of the tongue because of chorda tympani involvement.

Treatment of Bell's palsy is symptomatic and supportive. The most important consideration is care of the cornea when the patient cannot voluntarily close the affected eye. Important procedures are patching the eye and keeping it closed, particularly when the patient is asleep so that the bedclothes do not scratch the cornea, using artificial tears several times during the day, and training the patient manually to close the eyelid repeatedly to clear the cornea of dust particles. The cornea should frequently be observed to be certain that no ulceration has occurred. Simple massage following the normal pull of the involved muscle should be carried out repeatedly by the patient. When the mouth sags badly on the affected side, a hook device may be made to slip over the ear and to hold up the angle of the mouth on that side.

Usually there is considerable improvement, but it is a matter of weeks to months before recovery. Many patients stop short of a complete recovery. In these instances of partial recovery there may be a crossed regeneration of the fibers so that the fibers to the orbicularis oculi find their way to the orbicularis oris and vice versa. When the patient blinks his eyes, the corner of the mouth on the involved side twitches, and conversely when he purses his lips, the eyelid partially closes on that side. This is a useful sign to indicate that an old facial palsy is definitely peripheral and not central.

Eighth cranial (auditory) nerve

The most common disease of the eighth cranial nerve is **Meniere's disease,** which has its onset in patients in middle or later life. It is characterized by acute, sudden attacks of vertigo, either clockwise or counterclockwise, objective or subjective, and lasting a matter of minutes to hours, associated with nausea, vomiting, and unsteady gait. It may be severe enough to cause loss of consciousness. The first attack is difficult indeed to differentiate from labyrinthitis. The recurring attacks are characteristic of Meniere's disease, but they also reflect the possibility of the presence of an acoustic neurinoma. Patients with repeated attacks develop tinnitus and progressive deafness. Only the two parts of the eighth cranial nerve are involved. The other cranial nerves are spared. Definitive hearing tests show a progressive nerve deafness of the ear on the affected side. Caloric stimulation may reproduce one of the patient's attacks of Meniere's disease, but as the disease progresses the labyrinth on the affected side also becomes hypoactive.

The **treatment** of Meniere's disease revolves around the use of the antimotion sickness drugs and dehydrating agents such as chlorothiazide (Diuril) or the administration of potassium chloride with reduction of sodium intake. In some instances the administration of nicotinic acid is helpful. Surgical treatment may be necessary. Formerly this consisted of the intracranial section of the eighth nerve, but the modern approach is directed at the end organ itself. Since the pathophysiology of Meniere's disease is thought to be hydrops of the endolymph, various procedures have been devised for shunting or drainage. Other surgical procedures aim at partial or complete destruction of the end organ.

Tumors of the eighth cranial nerve are discussed on pp. 118, 121, and 122.

Ninth cranial (glossopharyngeal) nerve

The most important disease of the glossopharyngeal nerve is **glossopharyngeal neuralgia,** which usually occurs secondary to a nasopharyngeal lesion such as carcinoma of the tonsil. However, it may occur independently. Glossopharyngeal neuralgia consists of bursts of sharp, severe, lancinating throat pain that extends into the ear. The pain is precipitated by swallowing. The same medical treatment may be employed as for patients with tic douloureux. If medical therapy is unsuccessful, the glossopharyngeal nerve should be sectioned.

DISEASES OF THE PERIPHERAL NERVES

Under the term "neuritis" are included most nontraumatic diseases of the peripheral nerves. It is rare for true inflammation to occur in the peripheral nerves. Only in patients with syphilis, leprosy, and tuberculosis does this occur. However, by virtue of long usage the term "neuritis" is acceptable. **Mononeuritis** is a neuritis of a single nerve such as the ulnar, radial, or peroneal nerve. **Multiple neuritis** is an involvement of more than one nerve, for example, the ulnar and radial nerves. **Polyneuritis** refers to a symmetric involvement of many nerves, usually more pronounced distally and greatest in the lower extremities.

Polyneuritis or polyneuropathy due to vitamin deficiency

Polyneuritis or polyneuropathy due to vitamin deficiency may occur in patients with pellagra and other vitamin deficiency states and is most commonly seen in alcoholics with an impaired food and vitamin intake.

The **clinical picture** consists of pain, weakness, hyporeflexia, sensory changes, and later atrophy. The pain is both muscular and cutaneous, especially over the soles of the feet. Gentle stroking of the soles of the feet is excruciatingly painful. Slight to moderate squeezing of the muscles of the calves or thighs is equally painful. Patients have considerable distal weakness. When they are still able to walk, their gait becomes wide based with foot drop. Knee and ankle jerks are lost. A decrease in pain sensation occurs in stocking-glove fashion, beginning distally and gradually ascending about equally over the two lower extremities as one would draw on one's hose. The upper extremities are seldom affected until hypesthesia and analgesia in the lower extremities reaches about the middle third of the thigh. Then the same hypesthesia can be found beginning at the tips of the fingers and ascending in the upper extremities. When severe weakness has been present for several weeks, wasting of muscles occurs. There is no sphincter disturbance.

Therapy is directed toward an increase of vitamin intake (particularly the B complex vitamins and most particularly thiamine), physiotherapy, and the avoidance of alcohol.

Physical therapy in the early stages consists of the use of a cradle over the legs to keep the covers from pressing on the tender skin and muscles and from distorting the position of the legs. A footboard is employed to maintain the ankles and feet in good position to avoid contractures. Massage, passive and active exercises, and gait training are used as soon as possible.

Acute infectious polyneuritis

Acute infectious polyneuritis is also known by the synonyms Guillain-Barré syndrome, polyneuritis with facial diplegia, infectious neuronitis, and myeloradiculoneuronitis, to mention but a few. This disease can occur in persons at any age.

The **etiology** is thought to be on an autoimmune basis, and the development of a significant number of cases after swine flu inoculations furthers this concept.

Clinically this entity usually follows about two weeks after an acute upper respiratory infection. The onset is with weakness in the legs ascending in a matter of several days to involve the muscles of the trunk, upper extremities, and neck, the facial muscles, and occasionally even the extraocular muscles. Emergency treatment often becomes necessary because of the bulbar involvement, which may cause an inability to swallow and paralysis of respiration. The sensory levels develop the same as in patients with other polyneuritides. This syndrome can occur in patients with nonfaucial diphtheria and acute porphyria, may be simulated by tic paralysis, and as noted earlier, following inoculations.

The most important **laboratory test** for acute infectious polyneuritis is the examination of the spinal fluid. Characteristically the cell count is normal, the color clear, and pressure normal, but the total protein content is increased. This may be as high as 1,000 mg/100 ml. The elevation of total protein, however, may not occur at the onset and may require one or two weeks to become evident.

The **treatment** for patients with acute infectious polyneuritis consists of maintenance of an adequate airway, oxygenation when the airway is threatened, and the maintenance of nutrition during the bulbar phase. A respirator should be available for all patients with acute infectious polyneuritis until it is evident that respiratory involvement will not occur. The hospital staff must be well acquainted with the operation of the respirator. A tracheostomy set must be at hand, and someone qualified to perform an emergency tracheostomy must be available if these patients begin to pool secretions or develop cyanosis or tachycardia. Oxygen, when necessary, can be administered through the tracheostomy during the acute phase. Footboards may be used to maintain the feet in proper position, but it is better to make a thin plastic bivalve cast to hold the arms and legs in proper position to prevent contractures. Physical therapy should be instituted as soon as the disease has extended to its fullest course. Frequent evaluation of muscle power is indicated, since the return of function is not always symmetric and a permanent scoliosis and deformity could be caused by allowing the patient to be ambulatory while an asymmetric weakness in the trunk muscles still exists.

Neuritides of the nerve plexuses

Neuritides of the nerve plexuses are extremely uncommon. The most frequent form involves the **brachial plexus.** This was formerly seen as a sequel of serum sickness, but it may occur spontaneously. It is characterized by acute onset of excruciating pain in the shoulder and arm with tenderness of the plexus, in the supraclavicular fossa, and of the nerve trunks. The pain is so severe that the patient supports the extremity in a sling. Atrophy, discrete weakness, or discrete sensory loss may be permanent.

There are relatively rare but highly disabling instances of lumbosacral plexus involvement, appearing as predominantly if not exclusively femoral nerve in type. These may be due to trauma, vascular disease, or more frequently associated with diabetes. They are characterized by weakness of flexion of the thigh (iliacus and psoas muscle involvement) and weakness of extension of the knee (quadriceps weakness) with absent knee jerks. The onset is with excruciating pain, often resembling that of causalgia.

A rare form of neuritis is **chronic interstitial hypertrophic neuritis** (Déjèrine-Sottas disease, p. 209).

PRIMARY SCIATICA

Neuritis of the sciatic nerve occurs infrequently. **Clinically** there is severe pain along the sciatic distribution, with tenderness of the nerve, splinting of the affected leg, decreased or absent tendon reflexes, positive Lasègue sign, and hypalgesia in a dermatomal distribution. Spinal fluid protein level may be slightly elevated, but there is no radiologic, including myelographic, evidence of a ruptured intervertebral disk. **Treatment** is conservative, as described on p. 163.

MERALGIA PARAESTHETICA

Meralgia paraesthetica is a neuritis involving the lateral femoral cutaneous nerve. Since this is a purely sensory nerve, there are no motor signs. Clinically the patients complain of paresthesias over the anterolateral portion of the thigh. It is important to rule out pelvic tumors as the cause. This entity is common in pregnancy and disappears after delivery.

REFERENCES

Gurdjian, E. S., Thomas, L. M., Hodgson, V. R., and Patrick, L. M. L.: Impact head injury, G.P. **37:**78, 1968.

Kettel, K.: Peripheral facial palsy: pathology and surgery, Springfield, Ill., 1959, Charles C Thomas, Publisher.

Kitchen, C., and Simpson, J.: Meralgia paraesthetica: a review of 67 patients, Acta Neurol. Scand. **48:**547, 1972.

McCabe, B. F.: The surgical treatment of vertigo, Vertigo **3:**1, 1977.

Oester, Y. T., and Mayer, J. H.: Motor examination of peripheral nerve injuries, Springfield, Ill., 1960, Charles C Thomas, Publisher.

Williams, H. L.: Meniere's disease, Springfield, Ill., 1952, Charles C Thomas, Publisher.

13 Metabolic and toxic disorders of the nervous system

METABOLIC DISORDERS
Diabetes

The metabolic disorder most commonly causing involvement of the nervous system is diabetes. The usual **clinical picture** is that of a diabetic neuropathy. Absence of the Achilles and patellar reflexes in patients with diabetes is extremely prevalent and is considered by many to be evidence of early diabetic neuropathy. Diabetic polyneuropathy may be much more severe and resemble polyneuritis but is usually slow in onset and seldom of sufficient severity to involve the cranial nerves. Isolated diabetic neuritis of cranial nerves also occurs. Most commonly the sixth cranial nerve is involved. Neuritis of the lumbosacral plexus also occurs in diabetes. Adequate control of diabetes is helpful in alleviating the neuropathy, but a direct correlation between poor control of diabetes and the incidence of diabetic neuropathy does not exist.

Occasionally the neuropathy in patients with diabetes is so severe that it gives rise to a clinical picture resembling that of tabes. The diabetes may also produce a picture of combined system disease, but this is extremely rare.

Porphyria

Porphyria is a relatively rare disease that is probably caused by an inborn error of metabolism. The neurologic symptoms may be precipitated by the ingestion of sulfur-containing compounds, notably barbiturates.

Clinically the neurologic manifestations of porphyria include polyneuritis, abdominal pains, psychosis, and convulsions. The polyneuritis may closely mimic an acute infectious polyneuritis. The psychosis is an acute delirium. Convulsions are uncommon and do not occur as an isolated sign but are associated with the psychosis.

The predominant **diagnostic feature** of porphyria is the excretion of burgundy-red urine. The patient himself may be unaware of this, since the abnormal excretion is not constant. This is only irregular and is due to the presence of uroporphyrin in the urine. Allowing the urine to stand in light tends to darken it. The urinary determination of porphyrins is extremely helpful. It is important to note that even during an actual attack there may be a normal excretion of porphyrins. Therefore it is necessary to carry out repeated studies if the original urinary studies are negative and the disease is suspected.

Phenylketonuric oligophrenia

Phenylketonuric oligophrenia is a rather uncommon inborn error of metabolism responsible for mental deficiency. It occurs in the newborn infant. Unless it is diagnosed and treated within the early infantile period, it will give rise to permanent damage with severe mental retardation. The metabolic error is related to a failure to metabolize phenylalanine, the result of an absence of phenylalanine hydroxylase (fraction I) in the liver. This causes an interruption of the production of phenylketones. These phenylketones are spilled into the urine, and their presence can be detected by the use of ferric chloride and dinitrophenylhydrazine tests. It is important to test the urine of all newborn babies for phenylketones. When phenylketonuria is present, the child should be given a phenylalanine-free diet. Studies of families show that errors in the phenylalanine metabolism are present in other members of the family. This is therefore a familial disease.

Maple sugar urine disease

Maple sugar urine disease is a relatively rare inborn error of amino acid metabolism. The urine of children with this condition has a peculiar maple sugar odor and contains an accumulation of the amino acids—leucine, isoleucine, and valine. Significant deterioration occurs, with convulsions, paralysis, and other neurologic signs. These children die within a few months.

Other metabolic defects due to disturbances of amino acid metabolism producing mental retardation include the following: arginosuccinicaciduria and citrullinuria due to defects in the urea cycle; cystothioninuria due to a defect in the methionine-cysteine pathway; Hartnup disease due to a defect in the transport of tryptophan; and hyperglycinemia due to a defect in the breakdown of glycine and defects in proline metabolism. (Joseph's disease probably belongs in the latter category.) All of these types of amino acid deficiency are characterized clinically by mental retardation. Seizures occur in the proline deficiency group. Although these are all rare entities, where a sufficient volume of cases has been reported, genetic factors also play a role. Diagnosis of these diseases is made by careful biochemical studies of the blood and, more particularly, of the urine.

Galactosemia

Galactosemia is an inborn error of carbohydrate metabolism, in which patients fail to metabolize galactose. This, too, leads to severe mental retardation, cataracts, hepatosplenomegaly, and seizures. The disease is indicated by the presence of large amounts of galactose in the urine and high blood levels of galactose. Treatment consists in the substitution, usually of a soybean preparation, for galactose in the feeding formula of the newborn infant.

Spontaneous, or **idiopathic, hypoglycemia** is an uncommon disturbance of carbohydrate metabolism. This may be induced in some patients by casein or L-leucine administration. Convulsive seizures are a prominent part of the clinical picture, and mental defects may result from damage to the central nervous system caused by hypoglycemia.

Moderate mental retardation and hypoglycemic symptoms occur in patients with intolerance to fructose. This disease has a genetic basis. The biochemical defect is primarily deficiency of 1-phosphofructaldolase or secondary to a deficiency of phosphoglucomutase.

Encephalopathy also occurs in patients undergoing renal dialysis for many years. The encephalopathy results in slurred speech, myoclonic jerks of the extremities, confusion and dementia, and eventually death.

LIPOIDOSIS—DISTURBANCES OF LIPID METABOLISM

The lipoidoses are diseases characterized by abnormal depositions of the various lipids within the cells of the central nervous system. The lipids of the nervous tissue are classified by Folch-Pi and Sperry into (1) cholesterol, usually in the free form; (2) the phospholipids, which include lecithin, the cephalins, the phosphoinositides, and the phosphosphingocides; and (3) the glycolipids, which in turn include cerebrosides and gangliosides.

Xanthomatosis cranii, or Hand-Schüller-Christian disease, is due to a disturbance of cholesterol metabolism. This occurs in children, a little more commonly in boys than in girls, and is a hereditary disease. The characteristic triad of this disease is exophthalmos, diabetes insipidus, and radiologic evidence of involvement of cranial bones with extensive areas of rarefaction due to the presence of the xanthomas. The exophthalmos is caused by the involvement of the orbit. The only neurologic signs are those that are characteristic or significant of involvement by the bony destruction. This lipoid disease is treated by irradiation of the skull lesions. Diabetes insipidus may require specific therapy with vasopressin (Pitressin).

Cerebromacular degeneration (Tay-Sachs disease) is due to the deposition of abnormal fat in the neurons of the central nervous system. The abnormal fat deposited is a normal ganglioside (GM2), and the abnormal deposition is probably due to the absence of a specific hexosaminidase enzyme. This disease occurs most commonly in infants, but it may begin as late in life as puberty. It is more common in Jewish infants and affects either sex. There is a strong tendency for the disease to occur in more than one member of a family. Clinical features are blindness, mental deterioration, convulsive seizures that may occur when the patient is startled as well as spontaneously, pyramidal tract involvement with paralysis, and corresponding reflex changes.

Niemann-Pick disease is closely related to cerebromacular degeneration. The disorder is due to a disturbance of sphingomyelin metabolism and occurs only in infants. **Clinically** the picture is the same as that in patients with cerebromacular degeneration. The only distinguishing feature is a brownish discoloration in the skin and the presence of splenomegaly and hepatomegaly.

Gargoylism (Hurler's disease) is a relatively rare disorder occurring in infants and characterized by dwarfism, typical facial features (gargoyle), and hepatosplenomegaly. Blindness and mental deterioration are the other features of the **clinical picture.** The nature of the metabolic disturbance is not known but is thought to be a defect in mucopolysaccharide metabolism.

Posterolateral sclerosis

Posterolateral sclerosis has a number of synonyms. Combined system disease, subacute combined degeneration of the spinal cord, and radicular myelitis are the most common synonyms. Posterolateral sclerosis may be derived from a host of **causes,** but the most common one is pernicious anemia.

Etiologically posterolateral sclerosis due to pernicious anemia results from the failure to absorb vitamin B_{12} because of a somatic defect (of intrinsic factor) in the gastric mucosa. The lesions of the central nervous system consist of a spongy degeneration of the posterior and lateral columns of the spinal cord with demyelination of the posterior roots and the peripheral nerves.

The **clinical signs** usually become evident about the fourth decade of life. Since the lesions of the spinal cord are seldom symmetric, the clinical signs vary widely from patient to patient. Nevertheless, basically it consists of combinations of posterior column signs (loss of vibratory and position sense and ataxia) and corticospinal tract signs (spasticity, increased weakness, increased deep tendon reflexes, and positive plantar signs). The posterior root involvement leads to the loss of deep tendon reflexes.

The **diagnosis** is made not only on the basis of the clinical findings but also on the demonstration of the presence of anemia. Sometimes, however, the neurologic signs precede the frank appearance of the anemia. For this reason testing for free gastric acidity assumes great importance. The presence of free hydrochloric acid in the stomach usually precludes the diagnosis of pernicious anemia, even including a nonanemic phase. The radioactive cobalt vitamin B_{12} uptake studies serve as the ultimate confirmatory test. In very rare cases there is no anemia, and free hydrochloric acid is present in the stomach, but the B_{12} uptake studies determine that pernicious anemia is actually the cause of the combined system disease.

Treatment for posterolateral sclerosis is the same as for pernicious anemia, preferably with liver extract or vitamin B_{12} therapy. It is to be noted that the administration of folic acid does not prevent the development of neurologic signs and therefore is contraindicated. Vitamin B_{12} can be given in doses of 60 $\mu g/24$ hr intramuscularly for ten days and then once weekly. Thereafter one must be careful to monitor the peripheral blood for indications of control of the anemia. The weakness, which is secondary to the anemia, and the neuritic portion of the neurologic picture may be expected to disappear with adequate therapy, but once the posterior and lateral column signs are well developed, there is little hope for remission of these.

Hepatic encephalopathy

Hepatic failure may be accompanied by neurologic signs, which occurs regardless of the etiology of the liver disease and may therefore occur with acute virus hepatitis or chronic cirrhosis. **Clinically** the patient presents with mood changes and drowsiness, progressing into stupor and coma. Speech may be slurred, and a ''flapping'' tremor of the outstretched hands develops. Rigidity and muscle twitching also occurs.

Presumably the toxic effects are those of nitrogenous elements, especially ammonia, which has entered the systemic rather than the portal system probably because of anastomoses between the two systems.

Laboratory evidence of the nature of the disease is shown by increases in blood ammonia levels and by changes in the electroencephalogram. In severe cases the electroencephalogram shows delta waves with a triphasic component.

Treatment is aimed at reducing the absorption of nitrogenous substances, and this can be attained by severely limiting the protein intake and sterilizing the bowel with antibiotic agents. Serial electroencephalography can be used to monitor the success of therapy.

Reye's syndrome is an encephalopapthy associated with systemic fatty degeneration, including hepatic involvement, that affects infants and young children. It often follows viral illness and has an abrupt onset. Vomiting, confusion, hyperpnea, coma, and convulsions constitute the clinical picture. Hypoglycemia and abnormal liver function tests aid in the diagnosis. The mortality is about 90%.

DISORDERS DUE TO ALCOHOL

The disorders of the nervous system due to ingestion of alcohol basically are secondary to vitamin deficiency. Avitaminosis is most characteristically seen in abnormal drinkers, since they substitute alcohol for an adequate well-balanced food intake. However, many of these syndromes can occur in patients who are total abstainers from alcohol. An example of this is Wernicke's disease. The original description was of patients who suffered from vitamin deficiency because of an inadequate food intake secondary to an eschar of the esophagus.

Acute alcoholic intoxication is the development of deep anesthesia due to imbibing large amounts of alcohol.

Alcoholic paranoia is the development, in chronic abnormal drinkers, of paranoid trends, usually directed toward the spouse.

Alcoholic hallucinosis is also a sequel of chronic alcoholism. The hallucinations are usually in the auditory sphere and somewhat less commonly in the visual sphere.

Delirium tremens is an acute toxiclike psychosis with tremulousness, confusion, and wild uncoordinated behavior, marked by hallucinatory episodes, chiefly in the visual and auditory spheres. The visual hallucinations are bizarre as to size, shape, and coloring.

Korsakoff's psychosis also occurs in patients with chronic alcoholism. This is an organic mental defect with pronounced impairment of memory and even of orientation. Affect is usually flat, adaptable, and somewhat jovial. The outstanding characteristic of these patients is confabulation and ridiculous attempts to fill in the gaps for their memory lapses.

Pontine myelinosis occurs in alcoholism and also in other states of abnormal nutrition. It is characterized by long tract signs, especially corticospinal, and involvement of cranial nuclei. The definitive feature is that the signs are limited to pontine structures.

Wernicke's disease (polioencephalitis haemorrhagica superior) is a relatively rare disease due to capillary hemorrhages occurring in the hypothalamus (particularly the mamillary bodies), the nuclei of the third, fourth, and sixth cranial nerves, and the dorsal motor nucleus of the vagus nerve. **Clinically** patients with Wernicke's disease usually present with some neuropathy. In addition, they have extraocular muscle palsies and pupillary changes. The ocular manifestations are migratory and of varying nature. The examination shows considerable vasomotor disturbances, such as sweating and tachycardia, because of the lesions in the dorsal motor nucleus of the vagus nerve. These patients are tense and anxious and usually also have Korsakoff's psychosis.

The **treatment** of all the diseases due to alcohol includes the institution of vigorous vitamin therapy, the use of tranquilizing agents for the particular psychosis (for example, delirium tremens, hallucinosis, and paranoia), and the referral for proper psychiatric therapy to alleviate the underlying disorder causing the alcoholism.

The **prognosis** is extremely poor in patients with Korsakoff's psychosis and in those with alcoholic paranoia and hallucinosis. In patients with Wernicke's disease, if the acute crisis can be survived and the attendant Korsakoff's psychosis is not too severe, the prognosis is less grave. In patients with the neuropathies, the prognosis depends on the severity and duration of the problem. If the neuropathy has caused pronounced muscle wasting, the prognosis for full return of function is grave.

Alcoholic neuropathy, or polyneuritis (discussed on p. 174), is most evident distally—therefore in the lower extremities— and is due to vitamin deficiency.

TOXIC DISORDERS

Some metallic elements are toxic to the nervous system. From the standpoint of incidence of these toxicities, the most important elements are lead and arsenic. Manganese is important in the specificity of its toxic reaction on the nervous system, but poisoning caused by this agent is rare.

Lead intoxication

Lead poisoning is the most common form of heavy metal intoxication occurring either industrially or at home. **Clinically** two main types of lead toxicities affect the central nervous system. There is a **peripheral neuropathy** that occurs especially in adults. It is usually motor in type and involves the nerves supplying the extensor muscles to a greater degree than those of other muscles. This is especially prominent in the upper extremities. There may be no sensory changes whatsoever with the neuropathy. In children, particularly, the nervous system manifestation of lead poisoning may be an **encephalopathy** with convulsions, increased intracranial pressure, and focal neurologic signs. This symptomatology often leads to a difficult differential diagnosis between brain tumor and lead encephalopathy.

The important **laboratory studies** reveal increased amounts of lead in the urine and feces. Spectroscopic examination gives evidence of increased amounts of lead in the blood. In children radiographic studies of the long bones show lead deposits in the epiphyses.

Therapy is aimed at the avoidance of further exposure to the toxic agent and the mobilization of lead, leading to its excretion. Care, however, must be exerted in this regard, for with any additional mobilization of lead the neurologic symptoms may definitely be augmented. The use of BAL is not too successful, since it may produce a toxic agent by combining with the lead. Chelating with calcium disodium versenate may lead to a combination with the lead, forming a water-soluble, relatively nontoxic compound that can be excreted by the kidneys. Urea therapy may be of some help in reducing the increased intracranial pressure.

Arsenic intoxication

Arsenic poisoning may be acquired on an industrial or domestic basis. **Clinically** the most characteristic neurologic picture is that of a painful peripheral neuropathy. The cranial nerves are susceptible to arsenic effects, especially the auditory nerves and, when the toxic agent is a pentavalent arsenical such as tryparsamide, the optic nerves. The involvement of nerves, both peripheral and cranial, is most commonly induced by the inorganic arsenical compounds, whereas the organic compounds more often affect the central nervous system, producing a hemorrhagic encephalitis with rapidly developing coma, convulsions, and death.

Pathologically arsenic encephalitis is characterized by multiple perivascular hemorrhages scattered throughout the central nervous system.

In the **treatment** of patients with arsenic poisoning, BAL is the drug of choice.

Manganese intoxication

Manganese intoxication usually occurs industrially but is extremely rare. The central nervous system manifestations are prominent, and there is development of dyskinesias, particularly of the parkinsonian type.

Mercury intoxication

Intoxication with mercury in the acute form presents with lesions of the mouth, gastrointestinal disturbances, and acute delirium. In the chronic forms severe neurologic disturbances occur with dyskinesias, tremors, pyramidal tract signs, and optic atrophy coupled with a toxic psychosis.

Carbon monoxide intoxication

Carbon monoxide intoxication occurs as the result of an accident such as faulty house flues or automobile exhaust systems or due to suicidal attempt. Characteristic of the acute stage is the cherry red skin with high methemoglobin in the circulating blood. Survival may be complicated by the development of neurologic signs, especially those of basal ganglia involvement, notably parkinsonism. Strangely this may not develop for a period of time—as long as a year after the intoxication.

Botulism

Botulism is due to the effects of the toxin from *Clostridium botulinum* and is the result of eating contaminated food. The toxin affects the myoneural junction. The symptoms are predominantly motor and usually begin with oculomotor paresis and progress to involve all skeletal muscles, but the neck muscles are particularly singled out by the toxin. Respiratory involvement is serious in this entity.

In tetanus, usually due to wound infection by *Clostridium tetani,* the exotoxin affects the central nervous system and produces spasticity, usually beginning with the jaw and face, becoming generalized and often so severe as to result in opisthotonus. Tetanic convulsions are prominent.

In diphtheria the exotoxin may cause mononeuritis, the most common of which involves the palate.

Organic solvents and other preparations

Some of the chemical solvents used in industry have toxic effects on the central or peripheral nervous system or both. **Carbon tetrachloride** may produce a potentially fatal encephalopathy from which severe residual and neurologic defects may result. **Carbon disulfite** may produce a parkinsonian-like syndrome or basal ganglia and cortical dysfunctions.

Trichloroethylene may cause a peripheral neuritis, mental changes, and even convulsions.

Triorthocresyl phosphate has been responsible for several epidemics of severe peripheral polyneuropathy with weakness, paresthesias, and pain, and even evidence of spinal cord damage. This has occurred when the toxic agent appeared as an adulterant in alcoholic beverages during prohibition (when the syndrome was known as ginger paralysis or jake paralysis). More recently triorthocresyl phosphate accidentally became an adulterant in the cooking oil market in North Africa.

Methyl alcohol, when accidentally ingested for ethyl alcohol, may produce optic atrophy, which may progress to complete blindness.

REFERENCES

Aronson, S. W., and Volk, B. W.: Inborn disorder of sphingolipid metabolism, Oxford, 1967, Pergamon Press.

Cumings, J. N.: Heavy metals and the brain, Springfield, Ill., 1959, Charles C Thomas, Publisher.

De Jong, R. N., and Magee, K. M. R.: Treatment of the metabolic and toxic disorders of the nervous system. In Forster, F. M., editor: Modern therapy in neurology, St. Louis, 1956, The C. V. Mosby Co.

Fleming, A. J., D'Alonzo, C. A., and Zapp, J. A.: Modern occupational medicine, Philadelphia, 1954, Lea & Febiger.

Garell, D.: Metabolic defects associated with mental retardation, Am. J. Dis. Child. **104:**401, 1962.

Gellis, S. S., Feinfold, M., and Rutman, J. Y.: Atlas of mental retardation syndromes: visual diagnosis of facies and physical change, Washington, D.C., 1968, Government Printing Office.

Glick, T. H., Ditchek, N. Y., and Salitsky, S.: Acute encephalopathy and hepatic dysfunction associated with chickenpox in siblings, Am. J. Dis. Child. **119:**68, 1970.

Huttenlocher, P. R.: Reye's syndrome: relation of outcomes with therapy, J. Pediatr. **80:**845, 1972.

Lyman, F. L.: Phenylketonuria, Springfield, Ill., 1963, Charles C Thomas, Publisher.

Menkes, J. H.: The pattern of urinary alpha keto acids in various neurological diseases, Am. J. Dis. Child. **99:**500, 1960.

Metabolic and toxic disorders of the nervous system. Proceedings of the Association held in New York, Assoc. Res. Nerv. & Ment. Dis., Proc. **32:**605, 1953.

Paguirigan, A., and Lefken, E. B.: Central pontine myelinolysis, Neurology (Minneap.) **19:**1007, 1969.

Swaiman, K. F., and Wright, F. S.: The practice of pediatric neurology, St. Louis, 1975, The C. V. Mosby Co.

14 Diseases of the muscles

MYASTHENIA GRAVIS

Myasthenia gravis is due to a biochemical lesion at the myoneural junctions, where there is a disturbance of acetylcholine formation and destruction. This is commonly thought to be the result of increased cholinesterase activity that interferes with normal transmission at the myoneural junction. Some evidence also shows that a circulating substance similar to curare may produce the symptoms. There is a growing indication that autoimmune processes may play a role in the disease process.

Pathologically the involved muscles are normal except that small collections of lymphocytes (lymphorrhagias) may occur in the affected muscles. Tumors of the thymus gland (thymomas) are present in some patients with myasthenia gravis, and in others hypertrophy of the thymus gland may occur. However, in the majority of patients the thymus gland is normal.

Myasthenia gravis is a disease primarily occurring in adult life and is more common in young adult women and in late middle-aged or older men. It may occur at any age and may even be present in the newborn; if the mother has myasthenia, it may be present in the infant. In these cases the symptoms remit in a matter of days. Rarely does the child himself have myasthenia gravis.

The **clinical picture** of myasthenia gravis is one of progressive weakness with exercise. The weakness is not generalized but occurs in one or more groups of skeletal muscles. The muscles most frequently involved in patients with myasthenia gravis are the extraocular muscles, the bulbar muscles of the jaw, tongue, face, larynx, and pharynx, and the axial or appendicular muscles. Repeated use of the affected muscles causes a progressive fatigue. With rest, muscle strength returns only to be weakened again by repeated use.

In the examination of patients with suspected myasthenia, the physician's interest is focused on the muscle groups under suspicion from the history, but it is important to check all muscle groups to document the exact distribution of the disease.

In testing for ocular movements, the eyes are kept in lateral or upward deviation or in convergence for a prolonged period, and progressive deviation of the eyes is noted. Subjectively the patient then notes diplopia. Ptosis, which may also develop during this procedure, can be accurately gauged as the lower border of the upper lid crosses the upper edge of the pupil.

Swallowing functions can be tested while the patient is eating. If documentary evidence is necessary, a repeated barium swallowing test can be monitored by fluoroscopy.

Truncal muscles can be tested by having the patient lie in the supine position on the examining table with arms folded across the chest and then having the patient repeatedly sit up and lie down. Normal individuals can do this without too much difficulty ten or twelve times before experiencing some fatigue. Myasthenic patients with truncal involvement show a progressive decrease in the degree to which they can erect the trunk, and they then begin to rotate to one side, using the shoulder to push up.

Repeated hand grips can be tested by having the patient alternately squeeze and release the examiner's fingers or the dynamometer. A presumptive diagnosis is made by the evidence of increasing weakness. In some patients, however, the increased weakness is slight and difficult to evaluate. This is more likely to be true of extraocular palsies. When the latter palsies are not consistent with any neurologic lesion, myasthenia should always be suspected.

The clinical impression gained by the demonstration of progressive weakness on exertion is enhanced by allowing the patient a short rest period and then demonstrating the return of function. The repeated elicitation at short intervals of the deep tendon reflexes in affected muscles shows a progressive decrease ending in areflexia. After a rest period the tendon reflex is again evident. This decrease to absence of muscle activity can be well demonstrated and documented by electromyography.

To establish the **diagnosis** firmly, a neostigmine or edrophonium chloride (Tensilon) test is performed. One milligram of neostigmine methylsulfate solution can be administered subcutaneously and the test for muscle strength repeated after 30 to 40 minutes. Tensilon can also be used as a test for myasthenia. Two milligrams are injected intravenously, and the patient is observed very closely for 1 minutes, since Tensilon acts within 20 to 40 seconds and its effect lasts only 1 minute. Another 3 mg can be given 1 minute after the initial injection, and after another minute, if necessary, an additional 5 mg, for a total of 10 mg.

Electromyography is of considerable value in establishing the diagnosis of myasthenia gravis. Rather prolonged tetanic stimulation reveals a progressive decrement in the amplitude of the evoked muscle potentials.

The **treatment** of myasthenia gravis consists of the development and maintenance of the proper dosage of anticholinesterase drugs. Neostigmine (Prostigmin bromide) can be given orally in 15 mg tablets or intravenously (Prostigmin methylsulfate). The dosage must be arranged for each patient to fit individual needs. Neostigmine frequently produces gastrointestinal symptoms, which may be counteracted by using atropine in doses of 0.5 mg either at the time of ingestion of neostigmine or 15 minutes before. Pyridostigmine bromide (Mestinon) in 60 mg tablets may also be used; this drug has the advantage of longer action.

The anticholinesterase drugs can produce weakness and a

crisis. It is clinically difficult and often impossible to ascertain whether the patient is in a myasthenic or a cholinergic crisis due to intoxication by the medication. A Tensilon test at this time is of great assistance, since the administration of Tensilon during a cholinergic crisis does not produce improvement in muscle weakness, indicating that the anticholinesterase drugs should be decreased in amount. In a myasthenic crisis, however, strengthening is noted during the Tensilon test. ACTH therapy may precipitate a myasthenic crisis, but if successful, it may help to control the disease with smaller doses of anticholinesterase preparations.

Surgical removal of the thymus is hazardous but, when successful, aids in controlling the disease. The ideal candidate for thymectomy is a female patient less than 25 years old who shows no evidence of a thymoma, who has had the disease for less than five years, and in whom there is inadequate response to medical therapy as well as a high relative lymphocytosis of the blood. Spontaneous remissions do occur, especially in pregnant women, although unpredictably.

MYASTHENIC SYNDROME

The clinical picture of myasthenia gravis may be closely mimicked by other disease processes, especially carcinoma of the lung and pancreas. Whereas the clinical picture in the individual patient simulates that of myasthenia gravis, ocular involvement is rare. Also the response to neostigmine is unsatisfactory. The diagnosis can be made by electromyography. With frequent stimulations the muscle responses become greater rather than diminishing, as is the case in true myasthenia.

PROGRESSIVE MUSCULAR DYSTROPHY

Progressive muscular dystrophy is a heredodegenerative disease, occurring in children and young adults, characterized by muscle weakness and wasting. **Pathologically** atrophy of muscle fibers occurs with destruction of striations, fatty degeneration, and homogeneity of the sarcoplasm. There are considerable variations in fiber size and central migration of sarcolemmal nuclei, with enlargement and vacuolization of these nuclei.

Clinically the disease affects children and young adults, being usually far more common in males than in females. It is possible that women transmit the disease. This disease can be further subdivided clinically according to mode of inheritance, sex of patient, distribution of the muscle involvement, and severity of the process.

The **Duchenne type,** or **pseudohypertrophic muscular dystrophy,** is X linked and affects only males. The onset is usually by the age of 3 years, and the first indication is difficulty with gait, especially on climbing stairs. The disease begins with involvement of the pelvic girdle, but the shoulder musculature is involved later. This form of dystrophy is severe, and usually the child is unable to walk by the age of 10 years, contractures and skeletal deformities occur, and death generally occurs by the age of 20 years.

Early in the disease the affected muscles are often large and Herculean, usually because of fat and fibrous tissue rather than hypertrophy of muscle fibers. Cardiac musculature is also involved in this disease and often leads to cardiac failure.

The **Becker type** of dystrophy, likewise X linked, affects males but is more benign. The onset is later, between the ages of 5 and 25 years, and the course is often as long as an additional twenty-five years. Pelvic musculature is involved first and later the pectorals. Cardiac involvement is uncommon.

The **limb-girdle type** of muscular dystrophy affects either men or women, and in most instances is autosomal recessive in transmission. The involvement may affect either shoulder girdle or pelvic girdle first but usually eventually will affect both areas. The disease may be more benign in patients whose initial involvement is in the shoulder girdle.

The **facioscapulohumeral type** of muscular dystrophy (Landouzy-Déjèrine) is transmitted by an autosomal dominant mechanism, occurs in both sexes, and is usually evident by adolescence. This type affects primarily the muscles of the face, shoulder girdle, and upper arms. Myopathic facies are well developed in this form, with atrophy of facial musculature and a tapiroid mouth. Neck muscles, particularly the sterno-cleidomastoid and trapezius, are atrophied along with the other muscles in the distribution. Weakness is experienced primarily in the muscles of the shoulder girdle.

Distal muscular dystrophy is rare in the United States but apparently is not uncommon in Sweden. The inheritance is autosomal dominant, affects both sexes, and begins in middle life. The onset involves the small muscles of the hands and later those of the leg.

Ocular myopathy was previously referred to as progressive nuclear or external ophthalmoplegia. This, however, is now known to be a true myopathy involving the extraocular muscles. The course is slow with progressive weakness of the extraocular muscles, and ultimately the eyes may assume the cadaveric position. There is often weakness of other muscles, including those of the face and especially the orbicularis oculi.

Laboratory studies in progressive muscular dystrophy reveal disturbances of creatine and creatinine metabolism, with decreased excretion of creatinine and increased excretion of creatine and a low creatine tolerance. These changes are related to the amount of muscle destruction and are not causal. The increase in serum transaminase levels also represents destruction of muscles.

No specific **therapy** exists at present for progressive muscular dystrophy. The patient's treatment is largely supportive and comprises the use of physical medicine regimens to prevent contractures and obtain maximal use of the affected muscles.

MYOTONIA DYSTROPHICA

Myotonia is the persistent contraction of muscle tissue after the cessation of voluntary effort or stimulation. In myotonia dystrophica the myotonic response is coupled with muscular atrophy and systemic impairments. This is a hereditary disease, and the mode of transmission is autosomal dominant.

The **pathologic process** is one of muscle atrophy similar to that occurring in patients with muscular dystrophy.

The **clinical picture** is characterized by myotonia muscular atrophy, premature balding, cataracts, and testicular atrophy; the onset is usually in middle life. The muscular atrophy affects the facial and scapulohumeral muscles and also the distal muscles of the extremities, especially the upper ones. The onset of the atrophy is generally preceded by the appearance of the myotonic reaction, which is characterized by an inability to release a firm grasp. The patient's fingers are literally peeled off the examiner's fingers. The same reaction can be demonstrated by holding the patient's hands with the palms up and briskly tapping the bulk of the adductor pollicis muscle. The thumb then is brought over slowly and maintained in adduction usually for 5 seconds or more. Percussing other muscles will produce characteristic bumps at the site of percussion. A tongue blade placed across the tongue and briskly tapped with a reflex hammer produces a myotonic contraction evidenced by a constricting band across the tongue at the point of impact. Cataracts are characteristic and occur in the posterior capsule of the lens. The balding is largely frontal and patchy. Because of the testicular atrophy, sterility occurs.

There is no specific **treatment** for myotonia dystrophica. No therapy alleviates the dystrophic or systemic aspects of this disease. Various medications have been used to alleviate the myotonic reactions. Quinine, prednisone, procainamide, and phenytoin have each shown some success.

MYOTONIA CONGENITA (THOMSEN'S DISEASE)

Myotonia congenita is a rare familial disease, which is evident at birth or shortly afterward. It may appear in a later period of life, often around puberty, and men are affected predominantly. The muscular disturbance in patients with myotonia congenita is characterized by the inability to begin contraction after the muscle has been at rest. Children find it difficult to stand suddenly and walk or to suddenly release objects held in the hands. With repeated movements normal facility appears. The myotonia is made worse by cold and improved by heat. This disease is closely related to myotonia atrophica.

PARAMYOTONIA CONGENITA

In paramyotonia congenita the myotonic response occurs only on exposure to cold. Patients also suffer attacks of muscular weakness similar to those seen in familiar periodic paralysis.

AMYOTONIA CONGENITA

Amyotonia congenita is a rare disease, occurring in newborn infants and characterized by a pronounced loss of muscle tone. This is one of the entities included in the category of "floppy" infant.

COLLAGENOUS DISEASES OF MUSCLE

Polymyositis occurs usually in adults, as a manifestation of collagenous disease and involves the proximal muscles symmetrically. There is an associated leukocytosis and increased sedimentation rate. Pain occurs in the affected muscles, and they become edematous and doughy on palpation. Muscle biopsy is not a definitive laboratory study, since differentiating between muscular dystrophy and polymyositis is often difficult. The disease may be acute and, indeed, fatal within a few days, or it may be chronic over a period of years. In patients with acute cases visceral involvement is often associated.

Dermatomyositis is a collagenous disease involving both skin and muscles and occurring in persons of either sex at any age. The muscle involvement is usually symmetric and proximal. The musculature of the neck is often affected. Early in the course and muscles involved are soft and doughy but later become hard and fibrous and may atrophy. Joint contractures may be present. The skin lesions vary and may be erythematous, urticarial, or even chronically pigmented. Visceral manifestations may also be associated with this disease.

The collagenous diseases of the muscles are **treated** with steroids. Cortisone is the drug of choice. It is given orally and the dosage adjusted to the disease process. Some patients who do not respond to cortisone respond dramatically to prednisone.

MENOPAUSAL MUSCULAR DYSTROPHY

It is not certain that menopausal muscular dystrophy is a distinct entity. However, in women at the climacterium insidiously dystrophic changes and weakness in the proximal muscles occasionally occur. These changes seldom involve the muscles supplied by the cranial nerve nuclei. The **treatment** is the same as that for patients with the collagenous diseases.

CONGENITAL MUSCULAR HYPOPLASIA

Under the general term "congenital muscular hypoplasia" can be included amyotonia congenita of Oppenheim, the central core disease of Shy and Magee, and the cases described by Walton and others.

Pathologically no lesions of the central or peripheral nervous system occur. The skeletal muscle fibers may be predominantly small in size (Turner) or may present a condensation of basophilic material in the center of the muscle fiber (Shy and Magee), referred to as central core disease. In some cases, referred to as nemaline myopathy, rod-shaped bodies occur within the muscle fibers. Abnormalities of the mitochondria (mitochondrial myopathies) and myotubules resembling fetal muscle structure also occur but are uncommon.

Clinically, at birth the child is "floppy" because of the extensive hypotonia. There is also considerable weakness, which is greater proximally and is symmetric. Because of the weakness, these children often develop severe respiratory infections. If they survive these, there is a slow but progressive improvement in muscle strength but seldom to a complete development. Usually more than one member of a family is affected.

In the nemaline myopathies there are, in addition to the muscle weakness, prognathism, high arched palate, skeletal changes suggestive of arachnodactyly, and facial weakness. In the myotubular myopathies facial and extraocular muscles are also involved.

Carnitine deficiency can also produce a myopathy, since it facilitates the transfer of long chain fatty acids into the mitochondria of the muscle. The amount of carnitine ingested in insufficient for the demand, which is met by endogenously synthesized carnitine, accomplished by the liver. This rare entity should be suspected in children with unexplained myopathy and abnormal hepatic function or with muscle cramps and myoglobinuria.

The **treatment** is supportive and also includes the energetic treatment of pulmonary infections.

INFANTILE AMYOTROPHIC LATERAL SCLEROSIS (WERDNIG-HOFFMANN DISEASE: PROGRESSIVE INFANTILE MUSCULAR ATROPHY)

Infantile amyotrophic lateral sclerosis is a rare disease, probably occurring on a genetic basis. **Pathologically** there are changes similar to those in adults with amyotrophic lateral sclerosis (pp. 205 and 206).

Clinically this disease has its onset in about two thirds of the patients within the first 6 months of life. This entity, therefore must be considered in the differential diagnosis of the "floppy" infant. Pronounced weakness and hypotonia occur. Fasciculations are difficult to observe except in the tongue because of the abundant subcutaneous tissue in the infant. Usually the weakness is first noted in the trunk, shoulders, and pelvis.

The **prognosis** is poor in patients with this disease, and most affected infants die by the age of 2 years.

PAROXYSMAL MYOHEMOGLOBINURIA

Paroxysmal myohemoglobinuria is a rare disease characterized by episodes of polyneuritis similar to those of acute infectious polyneuritis (p. 175) and porphyria (p. 178). The attacks usually follow a febrile course, often associated with an upper respiratory disease. Urine is generally dark red in color and gives a positive benzidine stain. Proteinuria is common.

FAMILIAL PERIODIC PARALYSIS

Familial periodic paralysis is a rare disease characterized clinically by transient attacks of paralysis in the affected muscles, which are flaccid. These attacks begin distally in the lower extremities and progress upward but usually spare the respiratory and cranial muscles. This disease occurs predominantly in men and in more than one member of a family. The onset is generally in the second decade of life. The individual attacks may last for several hours to several days. Their frequency varies considerably; some patients have only several in a lifetime, whereas other patients are afflicted every several days. In some patients the attacks are precipitated by ingesting large quantities of food, especially carbohydrates.

The **etiology** of this disease is metabolic, and the attacks are related to a decrease in serum potassium. There is also a decrease in serum phosphate.

The **treatment** of patients with familial periodic paralysis is largely dietary, with avoidance of a high carbohydrate intake. Potassium salts are administered in an attack.

REFERENCES

Adams, R. D., Denny-Brown, D., and Pearson, C. M.: Diseases of muscle, ed. 2, New York, 1962, Paul B. Hoeber, Inc., Medical Book Department of Harper & Row, Publishers, Inc.

Bourne, G. H.: Muscular dystrophy in man and animals, New York, 1963, Hafner Publishing Co., Inc.

Desmedt, J. E., editor: New developments in EMG and clinical neurophysiology, Basel, 1973, S. Karger.

Eaton, L. M., and Lambert, E. H.: Electromyography and electric stimulation of nerves in diseases of motor unit: observations on myasthenic syndrome associated with malignant tumors, J.A.M.A. **161:**1117, 1957.

Greenfield, J. G., Shy, G. M., Alvord, E. C., and Berg, L.: An atlas of muscle pathology in neuromuscular disease, London, 1957, E. & S. Livingstone, Ltd.

Markesberry, W. R., McQuillen, M. P., and Procopis, V. G.: Muscle carnitine deficiency, Arch. Neurol. **31:**320, 1974.

Neuromuscular disorder. Proceedings of the Association held in New York, Assoc. Res. Nerv. & Ment. Dis., Proc. **38:**813, 1960.

Osserman, K. E.: Myasthenia gravis, New York, 1958, Grune & Stratton, Inc.

Proceedings of Third Medical Conference of Muscular Dystrophy Associations of America, Baltimore, 1955, The Williams & Wilkins Co.

Walton, J. N.: Disorders of voluntary muscle, ed. 2, 1974, Little, Brown & Co., Inc.

Walton, J. N., and Nattrass, F. J.: On the classification, natural history and treatment of the myopathies, Brain **77:**169, 1954.

15 Degenerative and heredodegenerative diseases of the central nervous system

DOWN'S SYNDROME (MONGOLISM)

Down's syndrome is a congenital disease characterized by mental retardation and a monogolian facial appearance. In many instances the disease is associated with a chromosomal abnormality—a trisomy of chromosome 21.

The mongolian facial appearance is produced by the round shape of the head and face and the slanting of palpebral fissures; often an epicanthal fold is present. In addition to these features, the children are hypotonic and have abnormal curvature of the little fingers, and the transverse crease of the palms is straight (simian).

Generally the mental retardation is severe. These patients are usually docile and amiable, but institutionalization is often necessary for their own protection. However, these patients tend to age prematurely, developing senile cataracts in early middle life and other stigmata of the aging process, including senile or presenile dementias. With the aging process the former docility is often lost, and patients become irritable and irascible.

NEUROCUTANEOUS DYSPLASIAS

Tuberous sclerosis is characterized by mental deterioration, convulsive seizures, and characteristic skin lesions. Pathologic lesions of this disease are widespread in neural and ectodermal tissue and are generally based on a maldevelopment due to a defect in germ plasm. Hard nodules occur on the surface of the brain and also within the cerebral substance. The latter may project into the ventricular system, where they can be visualized by pneumoencephalography. Sometimes the lesions are sufficiently calcified to be visible radiographically. The skin lesions are sebaceous adenomas in type and occur in a butterfly distribution about the nose. Other congenital tumors occur in these patients, including phakomas of the retina, which are readily visible on ophthalmoscopic examination. These children also have a high incidence of very rare tumors such as rhabdomyosarcoma.

Tuberous sclerosis is a rare disease, occurring sporadically and also on a heredofamilial basis and is a neurocutaneous dysplasia. The course is progressive, and the prognosis is poor in most patients, although occasionally the disease may halt. There is no specific treatment except that for the seizures.

Neurofibromatosis (von Recklinghausen's disease) is also a neurocutaneous dysplasia characterized by multiple skin lesions, neurofibromatous in type, occurring along the nerve distribution. Café-au-lait spots are common cutaneous manifestations. Neurinomas also occur in the spinal canal and on the cranial nerves, especially the eighth.

Sturge-Weber-Dimitri disease consists of angiomas occurring on the face (especially in the distribution of the first branch of the trigeminal nerve), cerebral cortex, and meninges. Angiomas also occur in the choroid layer of the eye. Vision may be affected, especially if glaucoma develops. Convulsive signs are common. Since the intracranial angiomas calcify, they are readily visible on radiographic examination.

Von Hippel-Lindau disease is discussed under the heading of hemangioblastoma of the cerebellum (p. 117).

CEREBELLAR ATAXIAS

Cerebellar ataxias are either primary or secondary. The **secondary ataxias** arise from chronic alcoholism or the presence of malignant neoplasms outside the central nervous system. Interest has been evoked by reports of cases of cerebellar ataxia with spasticity occurring in older patients and associated with a progressive hydrocephalus. The secondary ataxias are more common in men than in women and occur usually after the onset of the fifth decade.

Difficulty in coordination usually begins in the lower extremities, causing a disturbance in gait, due to intention tremor and ataxia. Later the upper extremities may be involved, and finally the patient may become dysarthric. Generally the cerebellum only is affected, and therefore no signs of the pyramidal tract or other systems appear.

The **primary cerebellar ataxias** also include a type which is similar to the secondary disease, in that it is limited to the cerebellum itself and the clinical features are identical. More commonly, however, in the primary forms other nervous system pathways are involved in addition to the cerebellum.

Friedreich's ataxia is the most common of the hereditary cerebellar ataxias. This is a degenerative disease of both the spinal cord and the cerebellum. The spinal cord lesions affect the posterior and lateral columns, including the dorsal and ventral spinal cerebellar tracts. Dorsal roots may also be involved. Friedreich's ataxia, too, is a familial disease. The onset is in the first or second decade of life. Certain anomalies are present, such as clubfoot, pes cavus, and scoliosis, and the onset is usually with gait incoordination. Gradually the upper extremities and truncal muscles become involved, and finally speech is affected. There is loss of vibratory and position sense, especially in the lower extremities, absence of knee and ankle jerks, and the appearance of Babinski's sign. Nystagmus usually develops rather late.

Hereditary cerebellar ataxia can also be combined with **spasticity** (Sanger-Brown and Marie). These cases begin later in life, usually after the fourth decade. Optic atrophy and involvement of the oculomotor nerves and nuclei are more common in the patients with cerebellar ataxia with spasticity.

Olivopontocerebellar atrophy is rare disease occurring in patients in adult or late middle life. It is similar to the other cerebellar ataxias, but more frequently it has combined with it basal ganglia features.

Differentiation between these cerebellar diseases is extremely difficult and is certainly mostly academic at this point.

Ataxia telangiectasia is a rare form of cerebellar ataxia, associated with telangiectasia of the mucous membrane and skin and sometimes associated with hypogammaglobulinemia. The disease begins in patients in childhood and is familial. Neurologic symptoms include progressive ataxia, choreoathetotic movements, pseudo-ophthalmoplegia, dysarthria, and decreased deep tendon reflexes. Intercurrent infection is often the cause of death. At postmortem examination the cerebellum is found to be atrophic.

AMYOTROPHIC LATERAL SCLEROSIS

Amyotrophic lateral sclerosis is a degenerative disease of the motor system occurring in patients in adult life and is relatively uncommon. **Pathologically** it is characterized by neuronal degeneration of the Betz cells of the motor cortex, of the ganglion cells in the cranial motor nerve nuclei, and of the ventral horn cells in the spinal cord. Demyelination of the corticospinal tracts also occurs. In the nomenclature, "lateral sclerosis" refers to the corticospinal tract demyelination, and "amyotrophic" describes the muscle atrophy due to the ventral horn cell degeneration.

The **cause** of this disease is unknown. Because of the peculiarly high incidence of the disease on Guam, it was at first speculated that genetic factors might be the cause. However, at present it is believed to be more likely that the high incidence among Guamanians is on a toxic basis and also that the Guamanian disease differs both clinically and pathologically from the traditional forms.

The **clinical picture** of amyotrophic lateral sclerosis depends on the location of the lesions. The degeneration of the ganglion cells of the cranial motor nerve nuclei produces bulbar palsy, characterized by voice hoarseness, dysphagia, dysphonia, and even complete aphonia. The cough loses its usual staccato quality, and there is difficulty in swallowing secretions and in clearing the bronchi. The tongue becomes atrophied and presents fasciculations.

The ventral horn cell lesions cause atrophy, loss of tendon reflexes, weakness, and fasciculations of the muscles, particularly those of the upper extremities and, to a somewhat lesser extent, of the lower extremities. The characteristic hand deformity in a patient with a well-developed case is described as a main en griffe, with curling of the fingers distally and extension proximally and wasting of the interossei muscles and of the eminences.

Degeneration of the corticospinal tract and of the Betz cells produces hyperactive deep tendon reflexes and plantar signs such as Babinski's and Chaddock signs. When the anterior horn cell signs are extensive in a particular extremity, the hyperreflexia of corticospinal involvement is masked, since the ventral horn cell is the final common pathway.

The **course** of the disease is relentless and progressive and has no known specific treatment. The usual duration is about two years, with rare cases lasting as long as twelve years. Supportive therapy may extend and improve life.

It is important in the differential diagnosis to be certain that the disease is not due to lesions of the cervical spinal cord, such as cervical osteoarthritis, ruptured intervertebral disk, or cord tumor. When bulbar signs are absent, it is important to rule out these other causes. Rarely, also, neurosyphilis (meningomyelitis) may closely mimic the clinical picture of amyotrophic lateral sclerosis.

PRIMARY LATERAL SCLEROSIS

Primary lateral sclerosis is a rare entity characterized by bilateral pyramidal tract signs beginning in late childhood or afterward. Certain cases, especially in children and young adults, are hereditary with a familial pattern. When these signs appear later in life without a positive family history, however, these patients over a period of time usually develop signs of other disease, such as amyotrophic lateral sclerosis, combined system disease, or cord tumor.

SYRINGOMYELIA AND SYRINGOBULBIA

Syringomyelia and syringobulbia combine in a rare disease, the **etiology** of which is probably heredodegenerative. This is due to the development of a syrinx, or cavity, in the spinal cord (syringomyelia) or medullar oblongata (syringobulbia) or both. The cavities in the spinal cord are in the cervical enlargement and less frequently in the lumbar enlargement. The cavities arise from a cystic degeneration of the cord. Demyelination about the cavity, gliosis, and progressive enlargement of the cavity occur.

Clinically these patients usually have some congenital anomaly, such as supernumerary nipples, facial asymmetry, or spade-shaped or otherwise peculiarly formed hands. Scoliosis may be caused by muscle weakness or occasionally by an anomaly of the vertebra such as a hemivertebra. The most characteristic clinical finding is that of dissociation of sensation, with loss of pain and temperature and preservation of light touch sensations. The most frequent area for this is in a shawlike distribution over the neck and shoulders and extending out into the upper extremities. Burns from cigarettes and heating pads are not felt and are only subjectively perceived because of the presence of a skin lesion. This may be the presenting sign. The loss of sensation is due to disruption of the pain and temperature fibers as they cross the median raphe of the spinal cord. As the cavity in the cord enlarges, the ventral horns become affected, with resultant atrophy, weakness, fasciculations, and loss of deep tendon reflexes in the extremities. Spontaneous pain is common and may be due to involvement of either dorsal root or tract. Pyramidal tract and posterior column signs appear as the syrinx destroys these pathways in the spinal cord. The onset is usually in the late teens. The course is slowly progressive but may be arrested. Bulbar involvement is indicated by the appearance of cranial nerve signs, such as involvement of the muscles of the palate, hoarseness of the voice, difficulty in protruding the tongue, and atrophy with fibrillations of the tongue. Respiratory disturbance may develop from the bulbar lesion. Charcot joints may occur in patients with this disease, more commonly in the vertebrae than in the extremities, although they may occur in either place.

The clinical picture of syringomyelia, particularly when the spinal cord only is involved, may be closely mimicked by an intramedullary spinal cord tumor, especially an ependymoma. This should be suspected especially when there is an absence of congenital anomalies.

Radiographic evidence of the syrinx consists of widening of the spinal canal. With myelography the shadow of the cord is seen to be increased in the transverse diameter.

Usually surgical **treatment** is of no avail unless the syrinx has caused an actual cerebrospinal fluid block. Then laminectomy and decompression are definitely indicated to preserve as much spinal cord function as possible. When there is any possibility of a neoplasm, surgical intervention is recommended to confirm the diagnosis. Opening of the cyst in most cases avails little or nothing, since the cerebrospinal fluid protein content within the cyst is the same as within the subarachnoid space, thus indicating continuity of cerebrospinal fluid pathways with the cyst. Radiation therapy is helpful in about one third of the patients. There is also a risk in radiation, since it may increase the rapidity of the disease process.

PERONEAL MUSCULAR ATROPHY (CHARCOT-MARIE-TOOTH DISEASE)

Peroneal muscular atrophy is a rare disease characterized by degenerative changes in the muscles, peripheral nerves, ventral roots, anterior horn cells, and posterior columns. There are usually hereditary factors, and other members of the family may also be affected. There may be an admixture with Friedreich's ataxia and other degenerative diseases of the skeletal muscles.

The onset is generally in the first or second decade of life. The disease usually begins in the lower extremities with wasting of the peroneal muscles and later of the calf muscles. As the gastrocnemius and peroneal groups are involved, the legs develop their characteristic storklike appearance. There are usually sensory changes, such as loss of vibratory and position sense in the lower extremities and impaired touch and pinprick sensation. The tendon reflexes, especially the ankle jerks, are lost early. If the quadriceps group is involved, as it usually is later, the patellar reflexes also disappear. This distal type of involvement also occurs in the upper extremities, and the disease may begin in the hands rather than in the lower extremities.

There is no specific treatment for the disease.

HYPERTROPHIC INTERSTITIAL NEURITIS (DÉJÈRINE/SOTTAS DISEASE)

Hypertrophic interstitial neuritis is a very rare heredofamilial disease characterized by proliferation of the interstitial tissue of the peripheral nerves leading to degeneration of myelin and loss of nerve fibers. The clinical picture is one of a chronic progressive polyneuritis.

This disease usually begins in patients in childhood or the late teens and in the lower extremities. It involves the distal parts and also the upper extremities. The characteristic clinical feature is a knobby, beaded feeling on palpation of the peripheral nerves. Diagnosis is confirmed by biopsy of a relatively unimportant nerve far distally in an extremity.

PRESENILE DEMENTIAS

Certain diseases of the cerebrum give rise to an appearance of senile psychosis in a period of life prior to the senium. The two most important of the presenile dementias are **Alzheimer's disease** and **Pick's disease.** Although clinically impossible to differentiate between these two entities, minor differences do exist.

Pathologically Pick's disease (lobar sclerosis) consists of atrophy of the frontal or temporal poles, whereas in patients with Alzheimer's disease the atrophy is more diffuse. Also the microscopic pictures differ. The senile silver-staining plaques (Alzheimer) are present in the cortex in patients with Alzheimer's disease.

The **etiology** of these diseases is unknown, but they tend to occur more frequently in some families.

The **clinical picture** in both diseases consists of an insidious onset with relentless progression and the appearance of an organic mental syndrome and disturbance in language function.

There is no treatment.

PROGRESSIVE SUBCORTICAL ENCEPHALOPATHY (BINSWANGER DISEASE)

Binswanger disease, of unknown etiology, is even more rare than the two preceding conditions.

Pathologically, in addition to arteriosclerosis, patchy areas of demyelination of the white matter appear in the cerebral hemispheres. Onset of the disease occurs in persons in the fifth and sixth decade of life. Intellectual impairment is the prominent symptom, but focal neurologic changes, including language defects, also develop.

OCCULT HYDROCEPHALUS

Occult hydrocephalus is an important entity to be considered in this chapter on degenerative and heredodegenerative diseases. Much of this importance lies in the response to treatment. Occult hydrocephalus has an insidious onset and exhibits a steady progression of signs of mental deterioration, cerebellar ataxia, and various movement apraxias. These signs are obviously readily confused, depending on which set of signs predominate, with the presenile dementias or the cerebellar ataxias. Diagnosis of occult hydrocephalus depends on laboratory testing–pneumoencephalographic evidence of some ventricular dilatation with diminished air over the cortex and intrathecal radioisotope scanning demonstrating a reflux into the ventricular system with decrease of flow over the cerebral cortex. The treatment consists of ventricular shunting.

REFERENCES

Crowe, F. W., Schull, W. J., and Neel, J. V.: A clinical and pathological genetic study of multiple neurofibromatosis, Springfield, Ill., 1956, Charles C Thomas, Publisher.

Greenfield, J. G.: The spino-cerebellar degenerations, Springfield, Ill., 1954, Charles C Thomas, Publisher.

Messert, B., and Baker, N. W.: Syndrome of progressive spastic ataxia and apraxia associated with occult hydrocephalus, Neurology (Minneap.) **16:**440, 1966.

Smith, R. A., and Norris, F. H.: Symptomatic care of patients with amyotrophic lateral sclerosis, J.A.M.A. **234:**715, 1975.

van Bogaert, L., and Cummings, J. N.: Cerebral lipidoses: a symposium, Springfield, Ill., 1957, Charles C Thomas, Publisher.

16 Congenital anomalies and defects of the nervous system

In view of the complexity of the nervous system and the complicated steps in its embryogenesis, congenital defects are surprisingly uncommon. Defects, when they occur, involve not only the nervous system but also the bone and even the skin covering.

Anomalies incompatible with life such as the **anencephalic monsters,** children in whom the forebrain has failed to develop and who seldom survive, are relatively rare.

Less drastic anomalies of the cerebral mantle and its connections include **congenital absence of the corpus callosum,** usually associated with some degree of hydrocephalus and mental retardation. Another anomaly is **agenesis** of one **cerebral hemisphere;** the other hemisphere usually appears normal. **Agenesis** of the **cerebellum** is also rare, may be unilateral or bilateral, and generally involves the lateral hemispheres.

Hydrocephalus may be caused by a congenital anomaly or may occur secondary to other diseases. A congenital anomaly may cause interference with the normal cerebrospinal fluid circulation, or the abnormality may affect the formation or absorption of cerebrospinal fluid. The obstruction to circulation within the ventricular system (noncommunicating hydrocephalus) occurs most commonly at the foramen of Monro, where the fluid leaves the lateral ventricle to enter the third ventricle, or at the aqueduct of Sylvius (congenital atresia of the aqueduct of Sylvius), or at the point of emergence of the cerebrospinal fluid from the fourth ventricle by way of the foramina of Magendie and Luschka (Dandy-Walker syndrome). A communicating type of hydrocephalus also occurs in which no demonstrable block of cerebrospinal fluid appears in the ventricular system.

Hydrocephalus may also be secondary to other diseases. As a sequela of meningitis, or toxoplasmosis, the same foramina, as well as the subarachnoid cisterns, may be occluded in the scarring process. Neoplasms of the brain stem or cerebellum may compress the ventricles or the aqueduct, and neoplasms arising from the choroid plexus within the ventricle may overlie the foramina.

The treatment of the obstructive type of hydrocephalus is surgical. A shunting procedure may be instituted; for example, one lateral ventricle is drained by means of an extracranial catheter into the cisterna magna. When this is not feasible in a patient with an obstructive hydrocephalus because of the location of the block or with a nonobstructive type of hydrocephalus, various drainage techniques are employed to empty the cerebrospinal fluid into the vena cava, left auricle, or body cavities. Valves may be employed to ensure a one-way flow.

Defects of closure of the neural tube and its coverings lead to cystic formations covered by skin, including cerebrospinal fluid and meninges, and with or without the presence of neural parenchymal elements. These may occur over the cranium (**encephalocele**) or over the lumbosacral region (**meningocele**). The latter is particularly likely to include nerve roots and, if sufficiently cephalad, portions of the spinal cord. It is then known as **meningomyelocele.**

Meningoceles are often associated with hydrocephalus (Arnold-Chiari syndrome). Children with lumbar or lumbosacral meningocele or meningomyeloceles frequently have weakness and sensory changes in the lower extremities and sphincteric disturbances.

Diastomyelia is a rare anomaly in which the spinal cord is divided longitudinally into two parts, usually at the point of a spur from the dorsal aspect of the body of one of the vertebrae.

Craniostenosis (Turmschädel or tower skull) is a premature closure of the sutures. The premature closure frequently involves the sagittal suture alone but may involve others. Craniostenosis may be associated with exophthalmos and protrusion of the lower jaw (Crouzon type). Children with craniostenosis can be treated by opening the cranium at or near suture lines and covering the edges of the bone along the apertures with a plastic to prevent rapid rehealing.

Cleidocranial dysostosis is the congenital absence of clavicles, combined with bony defects of the skull. This familial and is usually associated with neurologic problems, such as pyramidal tract signs and mental deficiency.

Porencephaly literally means a hole in the brain. This may be the result of a destructive lesion, usually vascular, and then may be further defined as encephaloclastic porencephaly. A similar defect may be due to failure of development, which is often referred to as schizencephaly. This form is bilateral and symmetric, whereas the encephaloclastic form is usually unilateral and, if bilateral, is asymmetric. Clinically in the encephaloclastic form the signs may be purely focal and depend on the location of the lesion. In the schizencephalic form, however, usually severe mental and neurologic defects are evident in very early life.

Lissencephaly is another failure of maturation in which the brain is small and there are no sulci over the convexities of the cerebrum. The brain therefore resembles that of a 3- to 5-month-old fetus. This condition presents clinically with microcephaly, convulsions, motor retardation, no response to environmental stimuli, and decerebrate posture. Minor other anomalies may be present.

REFERENCES

Courville, C. B.: Congenital malformations and anomalies of the central nervous system 1. In Pathology of the central nervous system, ed. 2, Mountain View, Calif., 1945, Pacific Press.

Daube, J. R., and Chou, S. M.: Lissencephaly; two cases, Neurology (Minneap.) **16:**179, 1966.

Henderson, J. L.: Cerebral palsy in childhood and adolescence, London, 1961, E. & S. Livingstone, Ltd.

Merrill, R. E., McCuthchen, T., Meacham, W. F., and Carter, T.: Myelomeningocele and hydrocephalus, J.A.M.A. **191:**21, 1965.

Woolam, D. H. M.: The effect of environmental factors on the fetus. J. Coll. Gen. Pract. **8:**35, 1964.

Yakovlev, P. I., and Wadsworth, R. C.: Schizencephalies, J. Neuropathol. Exp. Neurol. **5:**169, 1946.

Index

---

t after page number indicates table.

222 *Index*

Weight loss, 6
Werdnig-Hoffmann disease, 200
Wernicke's disease, 185-186
Western type of equine encephalo-
    myelitis, 139
"Wing-beating" movements, 104
Winging of scapula, 165
Withdrawal, drug, seizures after, 77

Wryneck, 105

X

Xanthomatosis cranii, 181

Z

Zarontin; *see* Ethosuximide
Zones, Hitzig's, 152